Geriatric Oncology

Guest Editor

RICHARD ROSENBLUTH, MD

CLINICS IN GERIATRIC MEDICINE

www.geriatric.theclinics.com

February 2012 • Volume 28 • Number 1

SAUNDERS an imprint of ELSEVIER, Inc.

W.B. SAUNDERS COMPANY
A Division of Elsevier Inc.

1600 John F. Kennedy Blvd., Suite 1800. Philadelphia, Pennsylvania 19103-2899

http://www.theclinics.com

CLINICS IN GERIATRIC MEDICINE Volume 28, Number 1
February 2012 ISSN 0749–0690, ISBN-13: 978-1-4557-3867-0

Editor: Yonah Korngold

Clinics in Geriatric Medicine (ISSN 0749-0690) is published quarterly by Elsevier Inc., 360 Park Avenue South, New York, NY 10010-1710. Months of issue are February, May, August, and November. Business and Editorial Offices: 1600 John F. Kennedy Blvd., Suite 1800, Philadelphia, PA 191023-2899. Periodicals postage paid at New York, NY, and additional mailing offices. Subscription prices is $257.00 per year (US individuals), $448.00 per year (US institutions), $131.00 per year (US student/resident), $334.00 per year (Canadian individuals), $559.00 per year (Canadian institutions), $355.00 per year (foreign individuals) and $559.00 per year (foreign institutions). Foreign air speed delivery is included in all *Clinics* subscription prices. All prices are subject to change without notice. POSTMASTER: Send address changes to *Clinics in Geriatric Medicine,* Elsevier Health Sciences Division, Subscription Customer Service, 3251 Riverport Lane, Maryland Heights, MO 63043. Telephone: 1-800-654-2452 (U.S. and Canada); 314-447-8871 (outside U.S. and Canada). Fax: 314-447-8029. E-mail: journalscustomerservice-usa@elsevier.com (for print support) or journalsonlinesupport-usa@elsevier.com (for online support).

Reprints. For copies of 100 or more, of articles in this publication, please contact the Commercial Reprints Department, Elsevier Inc., 360 Park Avenue South, New York, New York 10010-1710. Tel.: (212) 633-3812; Fax: (212) 462-1935, email: reprints@elsevier.com.

Clinics in Geriatric Medicine is covered in *MEDLINE/PubMed (Index Medicus), EMBASE/Excerpta Medica, Current Contents/Clinical Medicine (CC/CM),* and the *Cumulative Index to Nursing & Allied Health Literature.*

Printed and bound by CPI Group (UK) Ltd, Croydon, CR0 4YY

Transferred to Digital Print 2012

Contributors

GUEST EDITOR

RICHARD ROSENBLUTH, MD
Chief, Division of Geriatric Oncology, John Theuer Cancer Center, Hackensack
University Medical Center, Hackensack, New Jersey

AUTHORS

RICCARDO A. AUDISIO, MD, FRCS
Honorary Professor, University of Liverpool; Consultant Surgical Oncologist, St Helens
Teaching Hospital, St. Helens, United Kingdom

LODOVICO BALDUCCI, MD
Senior Member and Program Leader, Senior Adult Oncology Program, H. Lee Moffitt
Cancer Center & Research Institute, Tampa, Florida

MARUSCHA DE VRIES RN, BSN
Consultant, Cancer in the Elderly, Division of Care and Education, Comprehensive
Cancer Centre South Eindhoven; Participant, Program Geriatric Oncology, Netherlands,
Eindhoven, The Netherlands

MARTINE EXTERMANN, MD
Senior Adult Oncology Program, Moffitt Cancer Center, University of South Florida,
Tampa, Florida

TATYANA FELDMAN, MD
John Theurer Cancer Center, Hackensack University Medical Center, Hackensack, New
Jersey

ANDRE GOY, MD, MS
Chairman and Director; Chief Division of Lymphoma, John Theurer Cancer Center,
Hackensack University Medical Center, Hackensack, New Jersey

AVIAD GRAVITZ, MD
Resident in Surgery, Department of Surgery and Transplantation, Chaim Sheba Medical
Center, Tel-Aviv, Israel

SARAH HOFFE, MD
Assistant Member, Radiation Oncology Service Chief, Moffitt Cancer Center at
International Plaza, Tampa, Florida,

ARTI HURRIA, MD
Associate Professor and Director of Cancer and Aging Program, Department of Medical
Oncology, City of Hope Comprehensive Cancer Center, Duarte, California

DEEPAK KILARI, MD
Department of Medicine, Hematology/Oncology, James P. Wilmot Cancer Center,
University of Rochester, Rochester, New York

CARLO J. W. LEGET, PhD
Associate Professor, Ethics of Care, Faculty of Humanities, Tilburg University, Tilburg;
Associate Professor, Ethics of Care, University for Humanistic Studies, Utrecht, The
Netherlands

JANE JIJUN LIU, MD
Senior Adult Oncology Program, Moffitt Cancer Center, University of South Florida,
Tampa, Florida

ANTHONY MATO, MD
John Theurer Cancer Center, Hackensack University Medical Center, Hackensack, New
Jersey

SUPRIYA GUPTA MOHILE, MD, MS
Department of Medicine, Hematology/Oncology, James P. Wilmot Cancer Center,
University of Rochester, Rochester, New York

JOSHUA RICHTER, MD
John Theurer Cancer Center, Hackensack University Medical Center, Hackensack, New
Jersey

BENJAMIN ROSENBLUTH, MD
Chief, Department of Radiation Oncology, Holy Name Medical Center, Teaneck, New
Jersey

DAVID S. SIEGEL, MD, PhD
Chief, Division of Multiple Myeloma, John Theuer Cancer Center, Hackensack University
Medical Center, Hackensack, New Jersey

ARI VANDERWALDE, MD, MPH
Clinical Research Senior Medical Scientist, Global Development-Oncology, Amgen,
Thousand Oaks, California

ANDREW P. ZBAR, MD (Lond), MBBS, FRCS (Ed) FRCS (Gen), FRACS
Professor of Surgery, Department of Surgery and Transplantation, Chaim Sheba
Medical Center, Tel-Aviv, Israel

Contents

Cancer and Age: General Considerations

Sarah Hoffe and Lodovico Balducci

Cancer in the older person is increasingly common. The biological interactions of cancer and age are only partly understood. Management decisions in this population should be based on the natural history of the cancer, life expectancy, and the patient's tolerance of treatment. Financial and caregiver considerations are also important to assess. Cooperation between geriatrician and oncologists is essential. In France, this cooperation is already a reality that finds its expression in a network of units of oncogeriatrics distributed throughout the country.

Comprehensive Geriatric Assessment and Its Clinical Impact in Oncology

Jane Jijun Liu and Martine Extermann

More than 60% of cancer cases occur among individuals aged 65 and older, but older patients, particularly those with significant comorbidities, are undertreated and underrepresented in clinical trials. Whereas older cancer patients are increasingly receiving cancer treatment, determining treatment options can be difficult. Assessment tools and approaches have been adapted or developed to assist cancer specialists in the clinical management of older persons. This article reviews the literature along three lines: the ability of a comprehensive geriatric assessment (CGA) to identify unrecognized problems, the ability of a CGA to predict outcomes, and the results of implementing a multidisciplinary oncogeriatric intervention.

Management of Cancer in the Older Adult

Deepak Kilari and Supriya Gupta Mohile

This article summarizes the current literature linking cancer with aging. Discussion includes the potential mechanisms of development of cancer in the elderly, challenges in decision making, and the role of a geriatric assessment in formulating management options. This information will be of value to geriatricians, internists, and oncologists who manage elderly cancer patients.

elderly population, including cancer. We are therefore faced more frequently with the clinical problem of how best to approach the care of the elderly cancer patient.

THE CLINICS ARE NOW AVAILABLE ONLINE!

Access your subscription at:
www.theclinics.com

Preface

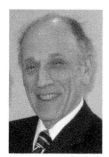

Richard Rosenbluth, MD
Guest Editor

It is time to revisit the subject of cancer in the elderly patient, the editors of *Clinics in Geriatric Medicine* have correctly decided. The advances in clinical oncology over the past several years have been truly dramatic. Biological therapy has improved overall response rates in a variety of cancers, and newer methods, "personalized medicine," designed to tailor therapy to individual patients promises to be a further advancement of significance.

All of this pertains especially to elderly people, who constitute the bulk of a clinical oncologist's daily practice. That the older cancer patient is different biologically, psychosocially, and functionally is now well-recognized in the medical community, as the subspecialty of Geriatric Oncology has finally taken its place among the other, more disease-oriented, subdivisions of oncology.

In this issue, we have gathered together a number of well-recognized specialists in various cancer fields who present to the reader the unique challenges they confront when treating older people. Beginning with a study of the biology of aging and a review of the current status of the comprehensive geriatric assessment, the principal tool in planning appropriate therapy for the elderly patient, our authors direct their attention to specific cancer types and modalities of therapy.

Breast cancer and the hematologic malignancies are common in older persons and, in part because of the wide array of treatment options now available to these patients, specific articles in these two areas are presented. The remainder of solid tumor oncology is covered in a separate article, as are the modalities of surgery and radiation therapy. A particular emphasis in all these articles is placed on how newer treatments can be of special benefit to geriatric patients by improving response and lowering treatment-related side effects.

Finally, an article on the ethics of treating elderly people highlights the often unperceived needs of the elderly and stresses the importance of responding to the unique desires and wishes of the geriatric patient rather than the all-too-frequent biases of the treating physician.

Clin Geriatr Med 28 (2012) ix–x
doi:10.1016/j.cger.2011.12.003
0749-0690/12/$ – see front matter © 2012 Elsevier Inc. All rights reserved.

geriatric.theclinics.com

We hope the articles herein presented will enrich the reader and give him a fuller appreciation of the special challenge as well as the unique gratification involved in treating the geriatric cancer patient.

Richard Rosenbluth, MD
Division of Geriatric Oncology
John Theuer Cancer Center
Hackensack University Medical Center
Hackensack, NJ 07601, USA

E-mail address:
RRosenbluth@humed.com

Cancer and Age: General Considerations

Sarah Hoffe, MD[a], Lodovico Balducci, MD[b],*

KEYWORDS

- Aging • Cancer • Chemotherapy • Management
- Prevention • Treatment

Cancer and age interact at several levels, including carcinogenesis, clinical presentation, prevention, and treatment. This article explores the interactions of cancer and aging from the viewpoint of the practitioner responsible of the care of the older person.

AGING AND CARCINOGENESIS

Age is a risk factor for most cancers (**Fig. 1**). By 2000, 50% of all malignancies occurred in the 12% of the population 65 and older; by 2030 one may expect 70% of all neoplasms in the older population.[1,2] Aging and carcinogenesis are connected through at least 3 mechanisms: Duration of carcinogenesis, increased susceptibility of older tissues to environmental carcinogens, and changes in body environment (chronic inflammation, increased resistance to insulin).[3]

The development of cancer involves multiple genomic and epigenetic changes over a prolonged time period.[4] The importance of the duration of carcinogenesis in increasing the risk of cancer in the elderly is revealed by the changing epidemiology of lung cancer. The median age of lung cancer is currently 71 years, up from 55 years 3 decades ago.[5] The lung cancer–related mortality is decreased by almost 50% in individuals younger than 65 and has increased at approximately the same rate for those 65 and over.[5] Smoking cessation is arguably responsible for these trends. Thanks to a decreased risk of cardiovascular deaths, the life expectancy of ex-smokers has become long enough for the development of lung cancer.[6,7]

Both experimental and epidemiologic studies reveal the increased susceptibility of aging tissue to environmental carcinogens. Tissues aging is associated with a number of carcinogenetic changes such as hypermethylation of antiproliferative genes, hypomethylation of oncogenes, point mutations, and chromosomal translocation.[8]

Authors have no professional or financial disclosures or conflict of interest to report, such as paid consultancy, stock ownership or other equity interest, or patent-licensing agreements.

[a] Moffitt Cancer Center at International Plaza, 12902 Magnolia Drive, Tampa, FL 33612, USA

[b] Senior Adult Oncology Program, H. Lee Moffitt Cancer Center & Research Institute, 12902 Magnolia Drive, Tampa, FL 33612, USA

* Corresponding author.

E-mail address: Lodovico.balducci@moffitt.org

Clin Geriatr Med 28 (2012) 1–18

doi:10.1016/j.cger.2011.09.001

0749-0690/12/$ – see front matter

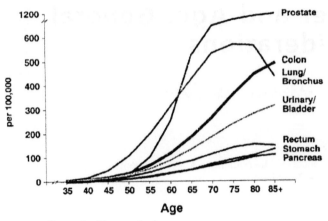

Cancer incidence rates in men.

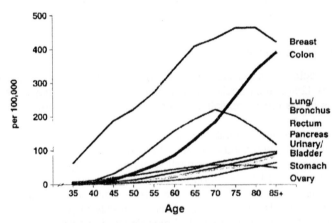

Cancer incidence rates in women.

Age-related incidence of selected cancers in men and women according to SEER.

Fig. 1. The increasing incidence of cancer with age. (*From* Yancik R, Ries L. Cancer in older persons: magnitude of the problem—how do we apply what we know? Cancer. 1994;74: 1995–2003; with permission.)

Aging tissues are in a condition of advanced carcinogenesis and are primed to the action of environmental carcinogens. The application of the same dose of carcinogen to the tissues of younger and older rodents causes more tumors in the aged animals.[9] Epidemiology suggests that the same is the case in humans:

- The incidence of prostate and colon cancer increases more rapidly with age, suggesting increased susceptibility of older tissues to environmental carcinogens.[9]
- The rate of malignant transformation of adenomatous polyps becomes more rapid with the age of the patient.[10]
- A dramatic increase in the incidence of certain tumors, such as non-Hodgkin lymphoma and malignant brain tumors has occurred in older individuals during the past 30 years.[11,12] Older people seem to develop cancer more quickly when exposed to new environmental carcinogens.

- Age is a risk factor for myelodysplasia and acute myelogenous leukemia (AML) after anthracycline treatment of breast cancer and lymphoma.[13,14]
- In a longitudinal study of the population of Bruneck, Italy, individuals with shortest leukocyte telomeres had more than a 3-fold increase in the risk of cancer with respect to those with the longest telomeres.[15] The telomere length may mirror of the functional age of a person.[16]

The clinical implications of these studies are 2-fold. First, elimination of environmental carcinogens is beneficial to older individuals. Second, older individuals may be primary candidates for chemoprevention that offsets the latest carcinogenetic stages.

Among the changes in bodily environments immune senescence, endocrine senescence, and proliferative senescence, as well as changes in body composition, may lead to more rapid neoplastic development. Decreased cellular immunity is associated with increased incidence of highly immunogenic neoplasms, such as lymphoma of the central nervous system.[17] The proliferative senescence of fibroblasts is associated with the production of tumor growth–stimulating factors.[18] Increased insulin resistance is common in the aged and is associated with increased circulating levels of insulin, a powerful tumor growth factor in the circulation. A recent experimental observation emphasizes the importance of insulin resistance in cancer development. The life span of rodents was increased by metformin treatment, which delayed the occurrence of cancer.[19]

Common changes in body composition include increase of fatty tissue and increased prevalence of male-type obesity. Both changes are associated with increased incidence of some cancers,[20] including cancer of the breast, large bowel, and prostate.

CLINICAL PRESENTATION

The natural history of cancer is critical to management-related decisions in individuals with limited life expectancy and reduced functional reserve.

Age and Tumor Behavior

The clinical behavior of some tumors changes with the age of the patient (**Table 1**).[21] Two important facts are highlighted:

Table 1
Clinical behavior of some tumors changes in older patients

Cancer	Clinical Behavior in the Aged	Mechanism
AML	More resistant to treatment	Increased prevalence of unfavorable genomic changes and of resistance to chemotherapy.
Non Hodgkin's lymphoma	Age is a poor prognostic factor	Increased circulating concentrations of interleukin-6 and increased risk of undertreatment.
Breast cancer	More indolent	Increased prevalence of hormone receptor rich tumors. Endocrine senescence.
Ovarian cancer	More lethal	Unknown.
Malignant brain tumors	More lethal	Increased prevalence of unfavorable genomic changes.

1. Some neoplasms become more aggressive and more lethal with aging; and
2. The change in tumors behavior involves at least 2 mechanisms: Changes in the tumor cells and in the tumor host.

The type of treatment received may also change with age and affect the outcome. Using a plant as a metaphor of cancer, the growth rate of the plant depends from the seed (the tumor cell), the soil (the tumor host), and the gardener (the provider).

Age is a poor prognostic factor for AML, owing to changes in the biology of the disease. These include higher prevalence of multidrug resistance, of unfavorable cytogenetics, and of NPM1 unmutated and flt3 mutated tumors.[22] At least in part, these changes may be explained by the fact that AML in older patients is preceded by myelodysplasia, which affects the early hematopoietic progenitors.

It is less clear why age is a poor prognostic factor for non-Hodgkin's lymphoma.[23] Increased circulating levels of interleukin-6, a powerful stimulator of lymphocyte replication, and other inflammatory cytokines may explain this finding.[24] Another possibility is inadequate treatment. In a systematic review of the management of large cell lymphoma, Lee and colleagues[25] demonstrated that individuals 60 and older had the same outcome as younger patients if they received the same dose intensity of chemotherapy. Dose intensity is the dose for unity of time (generally 1 week).

Metastatic breast cancer has a more indolent course in older women, with a higher prevalence of nonlethal bone and skin metastases in lieu of life-threatening visceral and brain metastases.[26] Veronesi and colleagues[27] reported that the risk of local recurrence after partial mastectomy at 5 years was 3% in women older than 55 and 19% in those 55 and younger, in absence of postoperative radiation therapy. The increasing prevalence of well differentiated, hormone-receptor rich tumors, combined with endocrine senescence that disfavor the growth of hormone-sensitive cancer, and the development of new and more effective forms of endocrine treatment may account for a more prolonged survival of older women with breast cancer.[26]

Age is a risk factor for early death in glioblastoma multiformis and malignant astrocytoma.[11] Poorer prognosis was associated with the overexpression of senescence-associated genes; that is, with advanced physiologic rather than chronologic age.

A recent observation suggests that the aggressiveness of some cancers may increase in the very old. It has been reported that prostate cancer diagnosed in individuals 85 and older was more likely to be poorly differentiated than the cancer diagnosed in younger individuals.[28]

Cancer Presentation in the Older Person

Three clinical aspects of cancer and age have elicited special interest: Cancer stage at presentation, prevalence and consequences of multiple malignancies, and general health of older cancer patients.

A number of studies[29] showed that the majority of cancers were diagnosed at a more advanced stages in older than in younger individuals. The reasons of delayed diagnosis may involve neglect of early symptoms of cancer, reduced utilization of cancer screening, and restricted access to health care.[30]

Multiple malignancies are seen in as many as 20% of cancer patients aged 70 and over.[31] The causes of multiple malignancies may include the following.

- *Field carcinogenesis*. Multiple neoplasms in the same tissue are more likely after the first, because all cells of that tissue have been exposed to the same carcinogens for the same time period

- Repeated imaging and laboratory tests to detect recurrence of a previous cancer may lead to diagnosis of a new neoplasm. The association of lymphoma and renal cell carcinoma may be partly explained by the use of serial computed tomography and magnetic resonance imaging of the abdomen.
- Previous cancer treatment may be carcinogenetic as in the case of chemotherapy-induced AML after previous cancer treatment.[13,14]
- Increased prevalence of indolent malignancies including prostate cancer and chronic lymphocytic leukemia in older individuals.

The history of multiple neoplasms does not seem to increase the risk of an older patient to die of cancer.[31]

At least 3 studies have shown that dependence in one or more instrumental activities of daily living (IADL) was as high as 70% and significant comorbidity was present in 40% to 90% of cancer patients aged 70 and older.[32-34] The prevalence of memory disorders, malnutrition, and dependence in one or more basic activity of daily living was present in as many as 20% of patients. When compared with an age-matched population without cancer, older cancer patients seemed to be in better health, although, with a reduced number of comorbid conditions and reduced prevalence of functional dependence.[33] The impression that cancer may be a disease of "healthy elderly" is reinforced by the low prevalence of neoplastic diseases among patients living in institution.[35] Thus, the majority of older individuals with cancer may benefit from cancer treatment if they have adequate medical and social support.

PREVENTION

Two preventative interventions may reduce the risk of cancer death: Chemoprevention and early detection of cancer in asymptomatic individuals.

Chemoprevention

Chemoprevention consists in the administration of substances that offset or block late carcinogenetic stages. Older individuals may represent ideal candidates for chemoprevention as older tissues may be primed to the action of late stage carcinogens. A number of substances prevent cancer in humans (**Table 2**).[36] The clinical use of these substances is controversial, however. Retinoic acid has serious complications and does not eliminate the genomic changes underlying cancer of the upper airways. The aromatase inhibitor exemestane is superior to the selective estrogen receptor modulators (SERMs) in preventing breast cancer.[37] Neither group of substances, however, have reduced breast cancer-related deaths, because they prevent only well-differentiated, indolent, hormone-responsive malignancies. Furthermore, both groups of medications are associated with menopausal symptoms and

Table 2	
Substances that prevent human cancers in clinical trials	
Medications	**Cancer Prevented**
Retinoic acid	Smoke induced cancer of the upper airways
SERMs: Tamoxifen, raloxifene	Breast cancer
Aromatase inhibitors: Exemestane	Breast cancer
5α-hydroxilase inhibitors: Finasteride, dusteride	Prostate cancer
Nonsteroidal anti-inflammatory agents	Cancer of the large bowel, breast cancer

debilitating arthralgias. Exemestane may cause osteoporosis, and SERMs deep vein thrombosis. It is legitimate to wonder whether regular screening mammography may not be a safer and less expensive way to reduce breast cancer-related mortality. The 5α-hydroxylase inhibitors reduce the incidence of prostate cancer but may increase the incidence of the most aggressive forms of the disease.[38] This treatment is associated with hot flushes, gynecomastia, and loss of libido. Although retrospective studies indicate that the regular use of aspirin decreases the risk of mortality for cancer of the large bowel, the optimal dose of the medication is unknown.[39]

Screening and Early Diagnosis

Randomized, controlled studies have demonstrated that early diagnosis of breast cancer with serial mammogram decrease the risk of cancer-related mortality in individuals aged 50 to 70 years; serial examination of the stools for fecal occult blood reduces the risk of mortality from colorectal cancer in individuals 50 to 80 years old[40] and serial screening for lung cancer with low-dose computed tomography reduced the lung cancer mortality in individuals 55 to 75 years old.[41] The information related to older individuals may only be obtained from retrospective analysis of clinical practices or may be inferred from studies related to a younger population. Analysis of the Surveillance, Epidemiology, and End Results data revealed that women aged 70 to 79 had a 2-fold reduction in breast cancer mortality if they underwent at least 2 mammographic examinations.[42-44] The benefit was present even in women with moderate comorbidity.[44] Because the initial benefits of cancer screening are seen 3 to 5 years after the initiation of the screening program, it seems reasonable to perform some form of screening for individuals with a life expectancy of 5 years or longer.

The value of some forms of cancer screening is controversial. This includes the use of serial prostate-specific antigen (PSA) determinations to screen asymptomatic individuals for prostate cancer, the use of serial Ca-15-3 determinations and transvaginal ultrasonography to screen asymptomatic older women for ovarian cancer, and screening for cervical cancer.

The most popular form of screening asymptomatic man for prostate cancer, serial assessment of serum PSA levels, has produced discordant results in 2 randomized, controlled studies.[45,46] In both studies, only individuals younger than 75 were included. The survival benefit of the positive European trial was marginal. The United States Preventive Service Task Force to recommend against screening men aged 75 and older[47] because the complications, discomfort, and cost of screening did not seem to be justified by the unproven benefits. These authors agree with the recommendation with a cautionary note. The recommendation is based on the assumption that local treatment of prostate cancer does not improve the overall survival of individuals 75 and older and is associated with substantial complications.[48] This tenet should be tempered by 2 facts. First, new forms of local treatment and, especially intensity-modulated radiation therapy (IMRT), have minimized the risk of therapeutic complications. Second, the life expectancy of the male population is becoming more prolonged and there is some new evidence that prostate cancer may become particularly aggressive and lethal in men over 85 years old.[28] Thus, is not impossible that in the future early detection of prostate cancer may become beneficial in an aging population. At present, there is no evidence that any form of screening for ovarian cancer is beneficial in women over the age of 50 years[49] or screening for cervical cancer is beneficial in those over the age of 60 who underwent regular screening at an earlier age.

Box 1
Cancer treatment

Locoregional forms of cancer treatment

  Surgery

  Radiation therapy

  Radiofrequency ablation

  Endoscopic tumor ablation

  Locoregional infusional therapy

  Systemic forms of cancer treatment

Hormonal therapy

  Cytotoxic chemotherapy

  Biological therapy

  Vaccines

  Cytokines

  Targeted therapy

TREATMENT

The various forms of cancer treatment are summarized in **Boxes 1** and **2** and **Table 3**. We review important recent advances in each form of treatment and thereafter discuss treatment-related decisions in older cancer patients.

Locoregional Therapy

Surgery

Age is a risk factor for early and late surgical complications and length of hospital stay.[50] The risk of surgical mortality and other complications is particularly elevated in the case of emergency surgery.[50] A number of advances both in anesthesia and in operative techniques have made surgery safer for older individuals. Of these, robotic surgery deserves mention, because it allows minimally invasive procedures.

Early diagnosis of cancer is particularly desirable as it may obviate the need of emergency surgery or of extended operations.[51,52] The operative management of metastatic cancer has become more common in recent years. Resection of liver metastases from cancer of the large bowel may be curative in 15% to 40% of cases.[53]

Radiation therapy

Radiation therapy is well tolerated, even by individuals of advanced age. New radiation techniques of special interest include stereotactic radiation therapy (referred to as radiosurgery if delivered in 1 fraction or as stereotactic body radiation therapy if more than 1 and up to 5 fractions), IMRT, image-guided radiation therapy, proton therapy, and brachytherapy.

Radiosurgery produces results comparable to surgery in the management of metastatic brain tumors, 3.5 cm in diameter or smaller.[54] In addition, it seems very promising in the management of many common cancers,[55-57] including cancers of the lung, liver, and pancreas. It is certainly indicated as an alternative to surgery in individuals who are poor surgical candidates. IMRT divides the beam into individual

---

Box 2
Hormonal therapy of cancer

Breast cancer

  SERMs

  • Tamoxifen

  • Toremifene

  • Raloxifen

  Aromatase inhibitors

  • Anastrozole

  • Letrozole

  • Exemestane

  Pure estrogen antagonists

  • Faslodex

  Estrogen

  Progestins

  Androgens

Prostate cancer

  Castration

  Orchiectomy

  LH–RH agonists

  LH–RH antagonists

  Estrogen

  Ketoconazole

  Androgen antagonists

  Abiraterone

"beamlets" so that higher doses can be delivered to the intended target and lower doses to the surrounding healthy tissues. It is currently the preferred form of treatment for localized cancer of the prostate and of the head and neck.[58] Advanced radiation technologies have incorporated imaging capability within the radiation delivery unit itself. This has resulted in image-guided radiation therapy, allowing for smaller treatment margins because the target can be verified with a daily image before turning the beam on. Brachytherapy consists of the administration of high doses of radiation in a localized area for a short period of time by directly placing radioactive sources adjacent or into the tumor target. It may be utilized for virtually all organs and most commonly is applied to cancer of the uterus, prostate, and breast (after partial mastectomy). The advantages of proton therapy include the sparing of normal tissue thanks to the rapid decline in dose from high-dose to low-dose region owing to the physical characteristics of the beam. Indications for proton therapy have historically been focused on cancers of the prostate as well as pediatric tumors; however, increasing access to this modality has fostered ongoing trials in cancers of multiple other sites.

Table 3 Targeted therapy	
Compounds	**Mechanism of Action**
Monoclonal antibodies	Immune destruction of the neoplasm: rituximab, ofatumumab, alemtuzumab
	Interference with neoplastic growth: trastuzumab, bevacizumab, cetuximab, panitumumab
	Immunoconjugates
	Stimulators of immune response: Ipilimumab
Small molecules kinase inhibitors	Cytoplasmic tyrosine kinase: Imatinib, nilotinib, desatinib
	Receptor-bound tyrosine kinase: Lapatinib, erlotinib, gemfitinib
	B-Raf kinase: Vemurafenib
	Multiple kinases: Sorafenib, sunitininib, pazopanib
Blockers of specific steps of the signal pathways	Mammalian target of rapamycin inhibitors
Reversal of epigenetic changes	Methylation inhibitors
	Isotone decarboxylase inhibitors
Others	Proteosome inhibitors
	Immune regulators: Thalidomide, lenalidomide

Radiofrequency ablation

This minimally invasive technique consists in destroying small tumors with microwaves administered trough a probe inserted in the tumor under radiologic monitoring or, more rarely, at the time of surgery. It has been used for the management of primary and metastatic tumors of the liver and the lung as well as for tumors of the kidney.[59] It is very safe, even for patients who cannot tolerate general anesthesia. The long-term effectiveness of this technique is not well known.

Endoscopic tumor ablation

Small, superficial tumors of the esophagus, bronchus, prostate, or bladder may be ablated endoscopically with phototherapy or cryotherapy. Phototherapy utilizes the high-intensity light of laser, cryotherapy involves deep freeze.[60] Endoscopic transanal resection of rectal cancer may allow organ preservation and is indicated in patients with small tumors or those who are poor surgical risks.[61]

Locoregional infusional therapy

This is mainly utilized for primary or metastatic liver tumors and may have 2 concomitant goals: The obliteration of the hepatic artery circulation supplying the tumor and the administration of cytotoxic chemotherapy or radioisotopes.[62-64] The hepatic artery is reached with catheterization of the femoral artery, and the complications of the procedure are negligible.

Systemic Cancer Therapy

Hormone therapy

The mainstay treatment of hormone-responsive breast cancer consists in the suppression of the estrogenic simulation of the tumor (see Box 1).[63] In postmenopausal women, the main source of estrogen is the aromatization of ovarian and adrenal steroids in the adipose tissue and in the breast. In the last few years, the aromatase inhibitors have become the preferred treatment of postmenopausal breast cancer both in the adjuvant and in the metastatic setting. A recent study showed that examestane is superior to raloxifen in the prevention of breast cancer.[37] The most serious complication of the aromatase inhibitors is bone loss. Concomitant treatment with bisphosphonates or other bone-sparing agents in indicated in women with osteopenia at the beginning of treatment. The SERMs were the preferred hormonal treatment of breast cancer before the aromatase inhibitors. Of these, raloxifen has been used only in the chemopreventative setting. The main advantage of the SERMs is that they prevent bone loss; the main disadvantage include rare but serious complications such as deep vein thrombosis and, in the case of tamoxifen and toremifene, endometrial cancer. Faslodex is a pure estrogen antagonist. As such, it does not cause the estrogen-like complications of SERMs (deep vein thrombosis, endometrial cancer).[65] In randomized, controlled trials it proved more effective than SERMs and anastrazole in metastatic breast cancer. Other forms of hormonal treatment, including estrogens in high doses, progestins, and androgens, are rarely used now. An ongoing study sought to establish whether treatment with estrogen reestablished the sensitivity to aromatase inhibitors in patients who have become resistant to those compounds.

The mainstay treatment of metastatic prostate cancer is androgen deprivation, which may be achieved with surgical or chemical orchiectomy.[66] Chemical orchiectomy is preferable because it allows intermittent androgen deprivation in patients with early metastatic cancer.[67] These patients may live several years and benefit from intermittent deprivation that minimizes complications, including loss of libido, osteoporosis, bone fractures, diabetes, coronary artery disease, fatigue, and anemia. Luteinizing hormone-releasing hormone (LHRH) analogs are presently the most common form of androgen deprivation. During the first month of treatment, it is advisable to combine the treatment with an antiandrogen, to offset the effects of the early surge of testosterone after the administration of the LHRH analogs. The main advantage of the LHRH antagonist is the lack of initial testosterone surge, but they are very costly. Ketoconazole blocks steroidogenesis very rapidly, but may lead to adrenal insufficiency and liver complications. This treatment is generally reserved to patients who experience a progression after treatment with LHRH inhibitors.

The antiandrogens are generally used in combination with LHRH analogs to offset the initial surge of testosterone. Some authorities recommend continuing the combination treatment beyond 1 month to neutralize the effects of the adrenal androgens. It is controversial whether a complete androgen blockade is superior to single blockade with LHRH analogs. Treatment with estrogen has been largely abandoned owing to the risk of fluid retention and deep vein thrombosis. Perhaps this was an unfortunate decision, because estrogens are not associated with some of the long-term effects of LHRH including loss of libido, osteoporosis, and hot flushes. Furthermore, the cardiovascular complications of estrogen were seen with 3 mg/d of diethylstilbestrol, whereas 1 mg/d may be sufficient. In addition to deep vein thrombosis and fluid retention, estrogen may cause painful gynecomastia, which is prevented with prophylactic breast irradiation.

Abiraterone is a very exciting new agent that is active in castration-resistant prostate cancer.[68] In addition to preventing the synthesis of androgen in the testicles and the adrenals, abiraterone blocks intratumoral synthesis of androgens that seems to be responsible for the majority of cases of castrate resistance. The experience with this drug is too initial to answer 2 of the major questions related to it: Is abiraterone able to prevent castrate resistance? May abiraterone be used as initial treatment of prostate cancer, in lieu of current treatment?

Cytotoxic chemotherapy

Cytotoxic chemotherapy is the mainstay treatment of most advanced neoplasms. It has been well documented that the risks of short and long-term complications of cytotoxic chemotherapy increase with age. The short-term complications include myelotoxicity, mucositis, cardiotoxicity, and peripheral neurotoxicity.[69] The long-term complications include myelodysplasia and acute leukemia, chronic cardiac dysfunction, and cognitive impairment.[69] As yet, it has not been clearly established whether cytotoxic chemotherapy is a risk factor for functional dependence and frailty.

A number of new advances have reduced the risk and increased the benefit of chemotherapy in older individuals. These include antidotes to chemotherapy related toxicity, predictive factors of response to chemotherapy, and methods to gauge response to chemotherapy early in the treatment course. Antidotes to chemotherapy toxicity include:

- Myelopoietic growth factors, for the prevention of neutropenia, neutropenic infections, and infection-related death.[70] Another major advantage of the use of these growth factors is that they allow the administration of chemotherapy in full dose and without delay, to guarantee the best outcome.
- Caphosol and keratinocyte growth factor for the prevention of mucositis. Caphosol is a supersaturated phosphate solution to be taken daily during treatment.[71]
- Dexrazoxane, an iron chelator for the prevention of anthracycline related cardiomyopathy.[71]

Genomic and proteomic have allowed to individualize the treatment of some tumors and hold the promise to for many other neoplasms. The development of several genomic profiles allowed to select patients that are more likely to benefits for adjuvant chemotherapy of cancer of the breast and of the large bowel. Of these, the most commonly utilized in the United States is Oncotype DX.[72]

Currently, the effects of cytotoxic chemotherapy in metastatic cancer are monitored by serial imaging or laboratory tests. In general, it takes at least 3 courses of treatment to establish whether a patient has benefited from chemotherapy according to these criteria. The serial measurement of the concentration of tumor cells in the circulation may allow to establish whether a response has occurred after the first treatment.[73] Thanks to that assay, many patients may not be exposed to unnecessary and potentially harmful doses of cytotoxics. The initial results in breast and prostate cancer seem to be very promising.

Biological therapy

A vaccine has recently been approved for the management of castration-refractory metastatic prostate cancer (Sipoleucel T), because it prolongs patient median survival of 4 months when compared with placebo.[74] The advantages of the vaccine include an almost complete absence of toxicity. The disadvantages include the complex preparation that involves 3 leukapheresis sessions. In addition, it is not clear how to monitor the patients because the vaccine does not produce responses detectable by serial imaging tests or assessments of the tumor marker (PSA).

The use of cytokines currently is very limited, especially in older patients. The main indications of high-dose interleukin-2 include malignant melanoma and renal cell carcinoma.

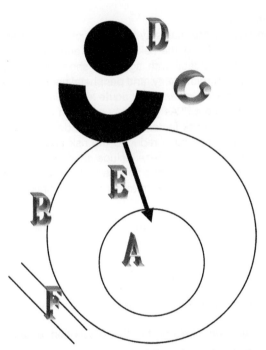

Fig. 2. Processes that regulate tumor growth. (A) Nucleus, that is the seat of epigenetic changes, such as DNA hyper and hypomethylation, histone decarboxylation, and micro-RNA. (B) Cell membrane. (C) Membrane growth factor receptor. (D) Growth factor. (E) Signal transduction cascade. (F) Neoangiogenesis

Targeted therapy

With this term, we refer to treatments that are directed against a specific tumor target (see **Table 3**) and promise to destroy the tumor with minimal damage to the host.[75] Using a military metaphor, targeted treatment would work as a missile, whereas cytotoxic chemotherapy works as carpet bombing.

Two types of targets have been studied: specific tumor antigens, and specific processes that control tumor growth (**Fig. 2**).[76] A detailed discussion of these processes is beyond the scope of the present article. The neoplastic cell has a number of growth factor receptors on the surface, which may be stimulated by circulating as well as paracrine and autocrine growth factors. The growth stimulus is transmitted to the nucleus through a cascade of molecular reactions in which tyrosine kinases play a major role. This cascade is a "check-and-balance" process that includes reactions aimed to suppress the tumor growth or to cause apoptosis, in addition to those that stimulate growth. In addition, tumor growth requires the formation of new vessels (neoangiogenesis). The tumor growth may result from a combination of the following changes.

- Inhibition of antiproliferative genes and overexpression of oncogenes. Some of these changes are epigenetic and may be reversible with new medications.
- Excessive production of growth factors or excessive expression of growth factor receptors. Of these the most typical is the overexpression of epidermal growth factor 2 (HER2neu) in very aggressive forms of breast cancer.

- Increased activity of reactions that stimulate tumor growth and decreased activity of those that inhibit it in the signal transduction cascade.

Some targeted treatments have had a major impact and deserve to be mentioned:

- The inhibitors of the cytoplasmic tyrosine kinase over-expressed in chronic myelogenous leukemia as a result of the Bcr/abl translocation—imatinib, nilotinib, and desatinib—have led to a prolonged control and possibly a cure in approximately 80% of cases chronic myelogenous leukemia. Allogeneic bone marrow transplant, which used to be the treatment of choice of chronic myelogenous leukemia, is reserved now for patients who become refractory to the medications. These oral preparations are generally well tolerated by patients of all ages.
- The monoclonal antibody trastuzumab is very active in the 25% of the patients with breast cancer who overexpress HER2neu. Older individuals are at increased risk for the cardiotoxicity, which is reversible in most of cases.[77]
- The monoclonal antibody rituximab is very active in all patients with B-cell lymphoma, and has prolonged the survival of patients with both follicular and large cell lymphoma. Except for the unusual occurrence of anaphylaxis, this treatment is well tolerated. There are some concerns that long term treatment may cause degenerative brain disease and immune suppression.
- Lapatinib, the inhibitor of the tyrosine kinase bound to the HER2neu receptor, is very active in patients with breast cancer who overexpress HER2neu. Of particular interest it is effective in patients whose disease progresses during treatment with Herceptin.[78] Except for diarrhea, it is also well tolerated.
- The immunomodulator lenalidomide is among the treatments of choice for multiple myeloma and early forms of myelodysplasia. It is also active in several lymphoid malignancies. It is associated with increase risk of thrombocytopenia and deep vein thrombosis.

Treatment-Related Decisions in Older Cancer Patients

The basic questions of cancer treatment in older individuals include life expectancy, treatment tolerance, social support, economic resources, and long-term consequences. Life expectancy is mainly important in the management of indolent malignancies, such as low-grade, early prostate cancer and low-grade lymphoma or in the administration of adjuvant (postoperative) treatment, whose effects may be seen only years later. Several methods based on geriatric assessment may be utilized for this purpose.[79,80]

The comprehensive geriatric assessment (CGA) may also be used to estimate the risk of complications of surgery and chemotherapy. The Pre-operative Assessment of cancer in the Elderly has been validated in 384 international patients aged 70 and over and has shown that dependence in one or more IADL and high fatigue score in the Brief Fatigue Inventory were predictive of surgical outcome, in addition to the American Society of Anesthesiology score.[81]

Two recent studies showed that the elements of the CGA may also predict the risk of chemotherapy related toxicity. In 500 patients aged 65 and older with different forms of cancer, Hurria and colleagues[82] created a predictive model of risk of chemotherapy-related toxicity based on age, type of cancer, chemotherapy dose, number of chemotherapy agents, hemoglobin levels, creatinine clearance, hearing deficits, falls in the last 6 months, dependence in IADL, and decreased physical and social activity (**Tables 4** and **5**).[82]

The risk score based on these elements was superior to the ECOG Performance Status as predictors of toxicity. The Senior Adult Oncology Program at the Moffitt

Table 4
Elements utilized for creating a predictive score

Elements	Score
Age ≥ 72 yrs	2
GI or GU cancer	2
Standard chemotherapy dose	2
Polychemotherapy	2
Anemia (hemoglobin < 11 g/dL in men and < 10 g/dL in women)	3
Creatinine clearance < 34 mL/min	3
Hearing loss	2
≥1 Fall in 6 months	3
IADL: Ability to take medications	1
Difficult to walk 1 block	2
Decreased social activity	1

Cancer Center in Tampa, Florida, also generated a predictive model called Chemotherapy Risk Assessment Score in High-Aged Patients [CRASH]; Extermann and colleagues, personal communication, American Society of Clinical Oncology Annual Meeting, Chicago, IL, 2010). According to this model, in addition to the type of chemotherapy, dependence in one or more IADL was a risk factor for hematologic toxicity and a Mini-Mental Status score of 24 or higher for nonhematologic toxicity. Although these models do need fine tuning, they demonstrate how the information of the CGA is essential in determining the risk of chemotherapy complications in older individuals. The CGA also provides important information on the socioeconomic status of the patient. "Financial toxicity" is a term adopted at the 2011 convention of the American Society of Clinical Oncology in Chicago, IL, to indicate how the cost of medications is a problem of access for many patients and, in particular, for older patients. The issues of the caregiver have not been studied as extensively in cancer as they have in dementia, but seem to be substantial. At the very least, it is important to ensure that the caregiver may be able to provide transportation to a health care facility on a short notice, supervise the patient's medications, and be readily available for any emergency.

SUMMARY

Cancer in the older person is increasingly common. The biological interactions of cancer with age are only partly understood and may provide some clues to future

Table 5
Score and risk of grade 3–4 toxicity

Score	Risk of Toxicity (%)
0–3	25
4–5	32
6–7	50
8–9	54
10–11	77
12–19	89

forms of cancer prevention and treatment. Management-related decisions in a population with limited life expectancy and limited functional reserve should be based on the natural history of the cancer, the patient's life expectancy, and the patient's tolerance of treatment. In addition, financial and caregiver considerations are important in assessing the treatment's benefits and risks.

Cooperation between geriatricians and oncologists seems to be essential to generate predictive models, as well as outcome information to improve the decision making in older cancer patients. It may also be essential in caring for a host of older cancer survivors. In France, this cooperation is already a reality that finds its expression in a network of units of oncogeriatrics distributed throughout the country.

REFERENCES

1. Smith BD, Smith GL, Hurria A, et al. Future of cancer incidence in the United States: burdens upon an aging, changing nation. J Clin Oncol 2009;27:2758–65.
2. Yancik R, Ries LA. Cancer in the older person. An international issue in an aging world. Semin Oncol 2004;31:128–36.
3. Balducci L, Ershler WB. Cancer and aging: a nexus at several levels. Nat Rev Cancer 2005;5:655–62.
4. Vineis P, Schatzkin A, Potter JD. Models of carcinogenesis: an overview. Carcinogenesis 2010;31:1703–9.
5. Edwards BK, Brown ML, Wingo PA, et al. Annual report to the nation on the status of cancer, 1975–2002, featuring population-based trends in cancer treatment J Natl Cancer Inst 2005;97:1407–27.
6. Crispo A, Brennan P, Jöckel KH, et al. The cumulative risk of lung cancer among current, ex- and never-smokers in European men. Br J Cancer 2004;91:1280–6.
7. Freedman DA, Navidi WC. Ex-smokers and the multistage model for lung cancer. Epidemiology 1990;1:21–9.
8. Gravina S, Vijg J. epigenetic factors in aging and longevity. Pflugers Arch 2010;459: 247–58.
9. Anisimov VN, Sikora E, Pawelec G. Relationship between cancer and aging: a multilevel approach. Biogerontology 2009;10:323–38.
10. Brenner H, Chang-Claude J, Seiler CM, et al. Case-control study supports extension of surveillance interval after colonoscopic polypectomy to at least 5 yr. Am J Gastroenterol 2007;102:1739–44.
11. Hoffman S, Propp JM, McCarthy BJ. Temporal trends in incidence of primary brain tumors in the United States, 1985–1999. Neuro Oncol 2006;8:27–37.
12. Han YY, Dinse GE, Umbach DM, et al. Age-period-cohort analysis of cancers not related to tobacco, screening, or HIV: sex and race differences. Cancer Causes Control 2010;21:1227–36.
13. Lyman GH, Dale DC, Wolff DA, et al. Acute myeloid leukemia or myelodysplastic syndrome in randomized controlled clinical trials of cancer chemotherapy with granulocyte colony-stimulating factor: a systematic review. J Clin Oncol 2010;28: 2914–24.
14. Gruschkus SK, Lairson D, Dunn JK, et al. Use of white blood cell growth factors and risk of acute myeloid leukemia or myelodysplastic syndrome among elderly patients with non-Hodgkin lymphoma. Cancer 2010;116:5279–89.
15. Willeit P, Willeit J, Mayr A, et al. Telomere length and risk of incident cancer and cancer mortality. JAMA 2010;304:69–75.
16. Houben JM, Giltay EJ, Rius-Ottenheim N, et al. Telomere length and mortality in elderly men: the Zutphen Elderly Study. J Gerontol A Biol Sci Med Sci 2010;66: 38–44.

17. Shultz TF. Cancer and Viral infections in the immunocompromised host. Int J Cancer 2009;125:1755–63.
18. Rodier F, Campisi J. Four faces of cellular senescence. J Cell Biol 2011;192:547–56.
19. Anisimov VN, Berstein LM, Popovich IG, et al. If started early in life, metformin treatment increases life span and postpones tumors in female SHR mice Aging (Albany NY). 2011;3:148-57.
20. Pais R, Silaghi H, Silaghi AC. Metabolic syndrome and risk of colorectal cancer. World J Gastroenterol 2009;15:5141–8.
21. Carreca I, Balducci L. Cancer chemotherapy in the older cancer patient Urol Oncol 2009;27:633–42.
22. Roellig C, Thiede C, Gramatzky M, et al. A novel prognostic model in elderly patients with acute myeloid leukemia. Results of 909 patients entered into the prospective AML 96 trial. Blood 2010;116:971–8.
23. Troch M, Wöhrer S, Raderer M. Assessment of the prognostic indices IPI and FLIPI in patients with mucosa-associated lymphoid tissue lymphoma. Anticancer Res 2010; 30:635–9.
24. Duletić-Nacinović A, Sever-Prebelić M, Stifter S. Interleukin-6 in patients with aggressive and indolent non-Hodgkin's lymphoma: a predictor of prognosis? Clin Oncol (R Coll Radiol) 2006;18:367–8.
25. Lee KW, Kim DY, Yun T, et al. Doxorubicin-based chemotherapy for diffuse large B-cell lymphoma in elderly patients: comparison of treatment outcomes between young and elderly patients and the significance of doxorubicin dosage. Cancer 2003;98:2651–6.
26. Carlson RW, Moench S, Hurria A, et al. NCCN task force report: Breast cancer in the older woman. J Natl Compr Canc Netw 2008;6(Suppl 4):S1–25.
27. Veronesi U, Ruini L, Del Vecchio M, et al. Radiotherapy after breast-preserving surgery in women with localized cancer of the breast. N Engl J Med 1993;318:1587–91.
28. Bechis SK, Carroll PR, Cooperberg MR. Impact of age at diagnosis on prostate cancer treatment and survival. J Clin Oncol 2011;29:235–41.
29. Goodwin JS, Osborne C. Factors affecting the diagnosis and treatment of older patients with cancer. In: Balducci L, Lyman GH, Ershler WB, et al, editors. Comprehensive geriatric oncology. London: Taylor and Francis; 2004. p. 56–66.
30. Terret C, Castel-Kremer E, Albrand G, et al. Effects of comorbidity on screening and early diagnosis of cancer in elderly people. Lancet Oncol 2009;10:80–7.
31. Luciani A, Balducci L, Multiple primary malignancies. Semin Oncol 2004;31:264–73.
32. Extermann M, Overcash J, Lyman GH, et al. Comorbidity and functional status are independent in older cancer patients. J Clin Oncol 1998;16:1582–7.
33. Repetto L, Fratino L, Audisio RA, et al. Comprehensive geriatric assessment adds information to the Eastern Cooperative group Performance Status in Elderly cancer patients. An Italian Group for Geriatric Oncology Study. J Clin Oncol 2002;20:494–502.
34. Ingram SS, Seo PH, Martell RE, et al. Comprehensive assessment of the elderly cancer patient: the feasibility of self-report methodology. J Clin Oncol 2002;20: 770–5.
35. Ferrell BA. Care of cancer patients in nursing homes. Oncology (Williston Park) 1992;6(2 Suppl):141–5.
36. Dunn BK, Greenwald P, Cancer prevention II: introduction. Semin Oncol 2010;37: 321–6.
37. Goss PE, Ingle JN, Alés-Martínez JE, et al. exemestane and breast cancer prevention in postmenopausal women. N Engl J Med 2011;364:2381–91.
38. Walsh PC. Chemoprevention of prostate cancer. N Engl J Med 2010;362:1237–8.

39. Rothwell PM, Wilson M, Elwin CE, et al. Long-term effect of aspirin on colorectal cancer incidence and mortality: 20-year follow-up of five randomised trials. Lancet 2010;376:1741–50.
40. Dunn BK, Greenwald P. Cancer prevention I: introduction. Semin Oncol 2010;37: 190–201.
41. National Lung Screening Trial Research Team. Reduced lung cancer mortality with low dose computed tomography screening. N Engl J Med 2011;365:395–409.
42. McCarthy EP, Burns RB, Freund KM, et al. Mammography use, breast cancer stage at diagnosis, and survival among older women. J Am Geriatr Soc 2000;48:1226–33.
43. Randolph WM, Goodwin JS, Mahnken JD, et al. Regular mammography use is associated with elimination of age-related disparities in size and stage of breast cancer at diagnosis. Ann Intern Med 2002;137:783–90.
44. McPherson CP, Swenson KK, Lee MW. The effects of mammographic detection and comorbidity on the survival of older women with breast cancer. J Am Geriatr Soc 2002;50:1061–8.
45. Andriole GL, Grubb RL, Buys SS, et al. Mortality results from a randomized prostate cancer screening trial. N Engl J Med 2009;360:1310–9.
46. Schroeder FS, Hugosson J, Roobol MJ, et al. Screening and prostate cancer mortality in a randomized European trial. N Engl J Med 2009;360:1320–8.
47. U.S. Preventive Services Task Force. Screening for prostate cancer: U.S. Preventive Services Task Force recommendation statement. Ann Intern Med 2008;149:185–91.
48. Bill-Axelson A, Holmberg L, Ruutu M, et al. Radical prostatectomy vs watchful waiting in early prostate cancer. N Engl J Med 2011;364:1708–17.
49. Buys SS, Partridge E, Black A, et al. Effects of screening on ovarian cancer mortality: the Prostate, Lung, Colon and Ovarian (PLCO) cancer screening randomized controlled trial. JAMA 2011;305:2295–303.
50. Katlic MR. Principles of geriatric surgery. In: Rosenthal RA, Zenilman ME, Katlic MR, editor. Principles and practice of geriatric surgery. 2nd edition. New York: Springer; 2011. pp. 235–52.
51. Shikanov S, Desai V, Razmaria A, et al. Robotic radical prostatectomy for elderly patients: probability of achieving continence and potency 1 year after surgery. J Urol 2010;183:1803–7.
52. Campos JH. An update on thoracic Robotic Surgery and anesthesia. Curr Opin Anesthesiol 2010;23:1–6.
53. Lupinacci R, Penna C, Nordlinger B. Hepatectomy for resectable colorectal cancer metastases: indicators of prognosis, definition of respectability, techniques and outcome. Surg Clin North Am 2007;16:493–506.
54. Stieber VW, Ellis TL. The impact of radiosurgery in the management of malignant brain tumors Curr Treat Options Oncol 2005;6:501–8.
55. Zimmerman R, Paulus R, Galvin J, et al. Stereotactic body radiation therapy for inoperable early stage lung cancer. JAMA 2010;303:1070–6.
56. Lo SS, Moffatt-Bruce SD, Dawson LA, et al. The role of local therapy in the management of lung and liver oligometastases. Nat Rev Clin Oncol 2011;8:405–16.
57. Minn AY, Koong AC, Chang DT. Stereotactic body radiation therapy for gastrointestinal malignancies. Front Radiat Ther Oncol 2011;43:412–27.
58. Gaspar LE, Ding M. A review of intensity modulated radiation therapy. Curr Oncol Rep 2008;10:2094–9.
59. Nour SG. MR guided and monitored radiofrequency tumor ablation. Acad Radiol 2005;12:1110–20.

60. Roscoe PA, Kucharczuc JC, Kaiser LR. Esophageal cancer in the elderly. In: Rosenthal RA, Zenilman ME, Katlic MR, editors. Principles and practice of geriatric surgery. 2nd edition. New York: Springer; 2011. p. 747–62.
61. Oliver AL, Ashley SW, Breen, E, et al. Neoplastic diseases of the colon and rectum. In: Rosenthal RA, Zenilman ME, Katlic MR, editors. Principles and practice of geriatric surgery. 2nd edition. New York: Springer; 2011. p. 889–906.
62. Mulcahy MF, Lewandowski RJ, Ibrahim SM, et al. Radioembolization of colorectal hepatic metastases using yttrium-90 microspheres. Cancer 2009;115:1849–58.
63. Arciero CA, Sigurdson ER. Diagnosis and treatment of metastatic disease to the liver. Semin Oncol 2008;35:147–59.
64. Balducci L. Treating elderly patients with hormone-sensitive breast cancer: what do the data show? Cancer Treat Rev 2009;35:47–56.
65. Robertson JF. Fulvestrant: how to make a good drug better. Oncologist 2007;12:774–84.
66. Flüchter SH, Weiser R, Gamper C. The role of hormonal treatment in prostate cancer. Recent Results Cancer Res 2007;175:211–37.
67. Shore ND, Crawford ED. Intermittent androgen deprivation therapy: redefining the standard of care? Rev Urol 2010;12:1–11.
68. de Bono JS, Logothetis CJ, Molina A, et al. Abiraterone and increased survival in metastatic prostate cancer. N Engl J Med 2011;364:1995–2005.
69. Balducci L. Pharmacology of antineoplastic medications in older cancer patients. Oncology 2009;23:78–85.
70. Shayne M, Balducci L. Hematopoietic growth factors in older cancer patients. Cancer Treat Res 2011;157:383–402.
71. Balducci L. Non hematologic complications of systemic treatment of cancer in the older-aged person. In: Naeim A, Reuben DB, Ganz PA, editors. Management of cancer in the older patient. Philadelphia: Elsevier Saunders; 2011. p. 127–33.
72. Kelly CM, Krishnamurthy S, Bianchini G, et al. Utility of oncotype DX risk estimates in clinically intermediate risk hormone receptor-positive, HER2-normal, grade II, lymph node-negative breast cancers. Cancer 2010;116:5161–7.
73. Lin H, Balic M, Zheng S, et al. Disseminated and circulating tumor cells: role in effective cancer management. Crit Rev Oncol Hematol 2011;77:1–11.
74. Kantoff PW, Higano CS, Shore ND, et al. Sipoleucel T immunotherapy in castrate-resistant prostate cancer. N Engl J Med 2010;363:411–22.
75. Gonsalves W, Ganti AK. Targeted anticancer therapy in the elderly. Crit Rev Oncol Hematol 2011;78:227–42.
76. Balducci L. Molecular insights in cancer treatment and prevention. Int J Biochem Cell Biol 2007;39:1329–37.
77. Serrano C, Cortés J, De Mattos-Arruda L, et al. Trastuzumab-related cardiotoxicity in the elderly: role of cardiovascular risk factors. Ann Oncol 2011 Aug 9 [Epub ahead of print].
78. Medina PJ, Goodin S. Lapatinib: a dual inhibitor of epidermal growth factor receptor tyrosine kinases. Clin Ther 2008;30:1426–47.
79. Lee SJ, Lindquist K, Segal MR, et al. Development and validation of a prognostic index for 4-year mortality in older adults. JAMA 2006;295:801–8.
80. Carey EC, Covinsky KE, Lui LY, et al. Prediction of mortality in community-living frail elderly people with long-term care needs. J Am Geriatr Soc 2008;56:68–75.
81. Pope R, Ramesh H, Gennari R, et al. Pre-operative assessment of cancer in the elderly: a comprehensive assessment of underlying characteristics of elderly cancer patients. Surg Oncol 2006;15:189–97.
82. Hurria A, Togawa K, Mohile SG, et al. Predicting chemotherapy toxicity in older adults with cancer. J Clin Oncol 2011;29:3457–65.

Comprehensive Geriatric Assessment and Its Clinical Impact in Oncology

Jane Jijun Liu, MD, Martine Extermann, MD*

KEYWORDS

- Comorbidity • Comprehensive geriatric assessment
- Cancer

In the last decade there has been an influx of clinical trials adopting comprehensive geriatric assessment (CGA) in oncology.[1–5] These trials can be categorized into three groups: (1) those focusing on recognizing unsuspected health problems, (2) those predicting treatment outcome and survival, and (3) those implementing multidisciplinary intervention–plan. In recent years the feasibility of implementing CGA in clinical trials was also a topic of research. Examples of some representative trials are summarized in **Table 1**. This article focuses on studies using a multidimensional geriatric assessment. Increasingly, short screening tools are used by oncologists to select who is in need of a multidisciplinary assessment. Interested readers can gain further information in the authors' recently published review.[17]

RECOGNIZING UNSUSPECTED HEALTH PROBLEMS

Studies profiling older cancer patients have now been conducted in several countries and settings and give us a fairly clear picture of the status of these patients (**Table 2**). Examples in this group include a prospective trial that was done in Korea,[6] where CGA data including comorbidity, activities of daily living (ADL), instrumental activities of daily living (IADL), cognition, psychological state, nutritional status, and medication were collected in 65 elderly cancer patients who were candidates for systemic chemotherapy. The trial reported that 25% of patients had a Charlson comorbidity index (CCI) score of 2 or more, 23% were ADL-dependent, and 14% were IADL-dependent. Using the Mini-Mental Status Examination (MMSE), it was found that 51% of patients had mild cognitive impairment (MMSE score 17–24), and 5% had cognitive impairment (≤16). A similar study[7] using the CGA questionnaire identified, out of the 245 elderly persons with cancer, that 49% required some assistance with IADL, 26% had Karnofsky performance scores lower than 70%, 21% reported at least one fall in

Senior Adult Oncology Program, Moffitt Cancer Center, University of South Florida, 12902 Magnolia Drive, Tampa, FL 33612, USA
* Corresponding author.
E-mail address: martine.extermann@moffitt.org

Clin Geriatr Med 28 (2012) 19–31
doi:10.1016/j.cger.2011.10.001
0749-0690/12/$ – see front matter © 2012 Elsevier Inc. All rights reserved.

Table 1
Examples of clinical trials incorporating or evaluating CGA

Type of Study	Article	Population	Study Design	Results/Conclusion
CGA detects unsuspected health problems	Kim, 2010[6]	Chemotherapy recipients, N = 65	Prospective, descriptive	CGA was feasible and could detect multiple unsuspected health problems including functional impairment and malnutrition in Korean elderly cancer patients receiving chemotherapy.
	Hurria, 2007[7]	Cancer patients, N = 250	Questionnaire	CGA questionnaire is feasible for use in the outpatient oncology setting and helped identify the needs of geriatric oncology patients.
CGA is prognostic	Winkelmann, 2011[8]	Lymphoma patients, N = 143	Prospective, observational	IADL and comorbidity were associated with survival.
	Arnoldi, 2007[9]	Outpatient cancer patients, N = 153	Retrospective	Frailty model identifies patients at higher risk of death.
	Clough-Gorr, 2010[10]	Breast cancer patients, N = 660	Prospective, observational	GA domains are associated with poor treatment tolerance and predict mortality at 7 years of follow-up, independent of age and stage of disease.
	Pope, 2006[11]	Cancer patients prior to elective surgery, N = 460	Prospective, observational	Preoperative assessment of cancer in the elderly represents a useful tool in evaluating oncogeriatric fitness for surgery.
	Kristjansson, 2010[12]	Electively operated CRC, N = 178	Prospective, observational	12% fit, 45% intermediate, and 43% frail; 7/21 (33%) of fit patients, 29/81 (36%) of intermediate patients, and 47/76 (62%) of frail patients experienced severe complications ($P = .002$).

CGA can predict response to treatment or change management	Tucci, 2009[13]	DLCL chemotherapy patients, N = 84	Retrospective	A comprehensive geriatric assessment is more effective than clinical judgment to identify elderly DLCL patients who benefit from aggressive therapy.
	Chaibi, 2010[14]	Cancer patients before receiving treatment, N = 161	Prospective, interventional	CGA significantly influenced treatment decisions in 82% of studied older cancer patients.
	Horgan, 2011[15]	GI/lung cancer, N = 30	Prospective, interventional	The impact of CGA in informing treatment decisions was modest and may be of higher value when the initial treatment decision is uncertain.
CGA is feasible	Hurria, 2007[7]	Cancer patients, N = 250	Questionnaire	CGA questionnaire is feasible for use in the outpatient oncology setting and helped identify the needs of geriatric oncology patients.
	Hurria, 2011[16]	Those enrolled in cooperative group cancer trials, N = 85	Questionnaire	CGA tool met the protocol-specified criteria for inclusion in future cooperative group clinical trials.

Abbreviations: CRC, colorectal cancer; DLCL, diffuse, large cell lymphoma; GA, geriatric assessment; GI, gastrointestinal; IADL, instrumental activities of daily living.

Table 2
CGA profiles of various oncogeriatric populations

Setting	Country	Age	ECOG PS 0-1 (%)	ADL-Independent	IADL-Independent	Depression	Cognitive Impairment	Comorbidity	References
Oncology outpatient	USA	75M	83.0	79	44	26 (GDS)	25 (MMSE <26)	94% (CIRS-G)/ 36% (Charlson)	Extermann 1998[18]
Oncology outpatients (VA)	USA	68m		31	42	14-26 (HADS)		5 (m, OARS)	Ingram 2002[19]
Oncology outpatient	USA	76m	74.0		51	21 (Distress Thermometer >5)		1.5 (m, OARS)	Hurria 2007[7]
Geriatric oncology outpatients	France	79M	60.0	58	46	53 (mini GDS)		94.7 (count)	Girre 2008[20]
Oncology outpatients, candidates for chemotherapy	Korea	71M	89.0	77	86	40	56 MMSE <25, 5 MMSE <17	25% Charlson ≥2	Kim 2010[6]
Oncology outpatient/inpatient	Italy	72M	74.0	86	52	40 (GDS)	37.8 (MMSE <24)		Repetto 2002[21]
Home health care	USA	77-78m				17-19 (Oasis)			Koroukian 2006[22]
Cooperative oncology trial	Italy	74M	81.0	85	33				Maione 2005[23]
Internal medicine/geriatric inpatients	Canada	79m		44	34		Mean MMSE 22		Retornaz 2007[24]
Oncology-acute care for elders unit	USA	74m		55	26	24	51 (clock)		Flood 2006[25]
Hospital-based cancer center	Canada	74.1M	83.9	89.3	65.2		24.1 (MoCa ≤26)	19.7% (FCI ≥4)	Puts 2011[26]

Abbreviations: ADL, activities of daily living; CIRS-G, Cumulative Illness Rating Scale-Geriatric; ECOG PS, East Corporative Oncology Group Performance Status Scale; FCI, Functional Comorbidity Index; GDS, Geriatric Depression Scale; HADS, Hospital Anxiety and Depression Scale; IADL, instrumental activities of daily living; M, median; m, mean; MMSE, Mini Mental State Examination; MoCA, Montreal Cognitive Assessment score; OARS, Older American Resources and Services Comorbidity Scale; OASIS, Outcome Assessment Information Set; VA, Veterans Administration.

the past 6 months, 94% had at least one comorbid medical condition, and 20% were underweight (body mass index <22.0).

Although these studies identify a large number of geriatric problems in cancer patients, many do not report in detail which problems were already known and which were detected by the CGA. Some data are nevertheless available. A pilot study assessed the ability of repeated CGAs to detect undiagnosed or undertreated problems in older breast cancer patients (median age 79) undergoing adjuvant treatment.[27] The patients underwent a multidisciplinary assessment by a nurse practitioner, pharmacist, social worker, dietitian, nurse, and geriatric oncologist in a geriatric oncology program at baseline, 3 months, and 6 months. An average of six unaddressed/underaddressed problems per patient were detected at baseline, and three new problems occurred over the following 6 months. Several studies report before and after treatment plans in oncology patients who were seen by a geriatrician.[14,28] The treatment changes were likely due in large part to the detection of significant unsuspected problems.

PREDICTING OUTCOMES

The prognostic and predictive role of CGA has been investigated in multiple studie (**Table 3**). Winkelmann and colleagues[8] reported a prospective trial with 143 patients newly diagnosed with malignant lymphoma who were evaluated by CGA including ADL, IADL, and comorbidities. In a Cox regression analysis, IADL (hazard ratio [HR] 2.1; 95% confidence interval [CI] 1.1–3.9) and comorbidity (HR 1.9; 95% CI 0.9–3.9) were independent and most strongly associated with survival time. Rather than studying the prognostic value of each component of CGA, Arnoldi and colleagues[9] synthesized the CGA parameters into an application model, which categorized the 153 cancer patients in an outpatient setting into frail, borderline, and nonfrail. 28.8% of patients were found to be frail or borderline. There was a significant difference in mortality between frail and nonfrail patients (*P*<.05), whereas there was no difference between borderline and nonfrail patients. A much larger longitudinal study[10] was done in 660 breast cancer patients, in which four geriatric assessment domains were described by six individual measures including sociodemographic by adequate finances, clinical by CCI and body mass index, function by number of physical function limitations, and psychosocial by the 5-item Mental Health Index (MHI5) and the Medical Outcomes Study Social Support Survey. Four measures representing all four geriatric assessment domains predicted mortality; these were inadequate finances (HR 1.89), CCI score at or below 1 (HR 1.38), functional limitation (HR 1.40), and MHI5 score less than 80 (HR 1.34).

Besides its prognostic role in medical oncology, preoperative CGA assessment of elderly cancer patients before elective surgery also showed similar effectiveness in evaluating oncogeriatric fitness for surgery and predicting perioperative complications in elderly patients.[11,12] At the 2011 American Society of Clinical Oncology annual meeting, Basso and colleagues[32] presented the results of a prospective cohort of older cancer patients who received a multidimensional geriatric assessment. Patients who were fit according to Balducci criteria had a 2-year survival of 83%, those who were vulnerable 70%, and those who were frail 60%.

CGA is not only prognostic, it is also predictive. Multiple trials have shown its potential in leading to change of medical management. Tucci and colleagues[13] analyzed a prospective cohort to assess whether CGA could identify elderly patients with diffuse, large cell lymphoma, who could be effectively treated with anthracycline-containing immunochemotherapy. In this study, according to CGA, 42 patients (50%) were classified as fit. These patients received curative treatment by clinical judgment.

Table 3
Prognostic and predictive role of CGA

References	Study Type	Cancer Type	IADL	ECOG/KPS	Other Predictors	Outcomes
Freyer 2005[29]	Prospective	Ovary, N = 83	Y	Y	Depression	Chemotherapy toxicity
			N	N	Depression, FIGO stage IV, nonoptimal surgery	PFS
			N	N	Depression, FIGO stage IV, >6 meds/day	OS
Wedding 2007[4]	Prospective	All, N = 200	Y	Y	Comorbidity	OS
Audisio 2005[30]	Prospective	All, N = 73	Y	Y	No. of comorbidities, GDS, IADL	30-d postoperative morbidity
Tucci 2009[13]	Retrospective	DLCL, N = 84			Balducci/Monfardini criteria	Frail patients had same prognosis whether or not treated by CHOP
					CGA-determined fit vs unfit	OS, PFS, RR
Extermann 2011[31]	Prospective	All, N = 518	Y	Y	LDH, diastolic blood pressure, MMS, MNA, MAX2 index	Chemotherapy toxicity (CRASH score)
Kristjanson, 2010[12]	Prospective	CRC, N = 178			Preoperative CGA-identified (fit, intermediate, or frail)	Rate of severe complication: 33% vs 35% vs 62%
Winkelmann 2011[8]	Prospective	Lymphoma, N = 143	Y	Y	Age (>60), ADL, comorbidity (3 or 4)	OS
Basso 2011[32]	Prospective	All, N = 880			Balducci frailty criteria (fit, vulnerable and frail)	2y OS 83%, 70%, 60%
Hurria 2011[33]	Prospective	All, n = 500	Partial	Y	Age, cancer type, Hb, CrCl, hearing, falls, decreased social activity, standard chemotherapy, polychemotherapy	Chemotherapy toxicity scores
Kanesvaran 2011[34]	Prospective	All, n = 249	N	Y	Age, nutrition (DETERMINE), GDS, stage	OS at 1,2,3 y (nomogram)

Abbreviations: CHOP, cyclophosphamide, doxorubicin, vincristine, prednisone; CRASH, Chemotherapy Risk Assessment Scale for High-Age Patients; CRC, colorectal cancer; CrCl, creatinine clearance; DLCL, diffuse, large cell lymphoma; ECOG, East Corporative Oncology group performance status scale; FIGO, International Federation of Gynecologists and Obstetricians for staging; GDS, Geriatric Depression Scale; Hb, hemoglobin; KPS, Karnofsky performance score; LDH, lactate dehydrogenase; MMS, Mini-Mental State; MNA, Mini Nutritional Assessment; PFS, progression-free survival; OS, overall survival; RR, response rate.

Their response rate (92.5% vs 48.8%; $P<.0001$) and median survival ($P<.0001$) were significantly better than those of 42 patients considered unfit by CGA. Among unfit patients, 20 had actually received curative intent therapy and 22 had received palliative therapy. The patients' outcomes were similar irrespective of the type of treatment received (median survival, 8 vs 7 months; P = nonsignificant). The authors concluded that a CGA is more effective than clinical judgment to identify elderly diffuse, large cell lymphoma patients who benefit from aggressive therapy.

IMPLEMENTING A MULTIDISCIPLINARY INTERVENTION

Multidisciplinary intervention studies follow essentially one of two schemes: randomized trials or prospective cohort evaluating the impact of an oncogeriatric consultation (**Table 4**).

Randomized Trials

At the 2006 conference of the International Society of Geriatric Oncology, Soejono and colleagues[38] presented the results of an Indonesian randomized trial of 87 older patients with stage III hepatocellular carcinoma randomized to either admission to the geriatric ward (which implemented interventions based on a CGA) or an internal medicine ward. At discharge, there was a significant improvement in the ability to complete ADL, as well as an improvement in pain and quality of life in patients who received care in the geriatric ward. Rao and colleagues[37] reported on a subset analysis of older patients with cancer who participated in a randomized study to evaluate the benefits of geriatric assessment and management units. Among the 99 patients with cancer, patients randomized to inpatient geriatric assessment and management units experienced improved pain control and mental health scores.

Two randomized studies evaluated the impact of incorporating elements of a CGA in the outpatient care of older patients with cancer who had undergone surgery. McCorkle and colleagues[35] published the results of a randomized study in which 375 patients (age range 60–92) with cancer who had undergone surgery were randomized to either a 1-month home intervention or usual postoperative care. The intervention consisted of home visits and telephone contact by an advanced practice nurse and included an evaluation of the patient's functional status, comorbidity, depressive symptoms, and symptoms of distress. On a stratified log-rank analysis, the patients in the intervention group had increased survival at median follow-up of 44 months (P = .002). A Cox proportional hazard model, adjusted for covariates including cancer stage and length of hospitalization, demonstrated that the relative risk of death for the control group was 2.04 (95% CI, 1.33-3.12, P = .001). This advantage in survival was evident among patients with advanced stage disease (67% intervention group vs 40% control group alive at 2 years). The investigators suggested that attention to the needs of patients and family and the monitoring of physical status and offsetting of early complications might account for this benefit. Another possible hypothesis is that this short intervention prevented acute deconditioning, which can lead to a protracted decline in physical function.

In a randomized study, Goodwin and colleagues[36] assessed the impact of nurse case management in the treatment of 335 older women with breast cancer. Patients in the intervention arm were more likely to have a return to normal functioning 2 months after completion of surgery and were more likely to feel that they had a real choice in their treatment decisions. Women with poor social support derived the greatest benefit from this intervention.[40]

Table 4
Clinical trials implementing a multidisciplinary intervention

Setting	Country	Intervention	Patients (No.)	Results	References
Discharged postoperative cancer patients	USA	Randomized: 1-mo home intervention vs standard of care	375	OS is not different in early-stage patients, but improved in intervention group among late stage patients.	McCorkle, 2000[35]
Postoperative breast cancer patients in community setting	USA	Randomized: 12-mo nurse case management care vs standard care	335	Patients in the intervention arm were more likely to have a return to normal functioning 2 mo after completion of surgery and were more likely to feel that they had a real choice in their treatment decisions.	Goodwin, 2003[36]
Early breast cancer patients, geriatric oncology clinic	USA	Pilot: Multidisciplinary CGA every 3 mo and interventions	15	Average 6 problems/patient detected at baseline, +3/patient over 6 mo. Average 17 recommendations/ interventions per patient. Interactions with cancer treatment.	Extermann, 2004[27]
VA inpatients and outpatients	USA	Randomized (subgroup analysis): geriatric vs medicine team	99	No difference in OS. The changes in the SF-36 scores for emotional limitation, mental health, and bodily pain were better for geriatric inpatient care cancer patients at discharge. No difference in QOL scores for outpatient care.	Rao, 2005[37]
Stage III HCC inpatients	Indonesia	Randomized: geriatric vs medicine ward	87	Greater increase in ADL & QOL, decrease in pain.	Soejono, 2006[38]
Academic hospital	France	Referral to geriatrician/ multidisciplinary treatment planning	105	38.7% of patients had a change in treatment plan.	Girre, 2008[20]

Academic hospital	France	Referral to geriatrician/ multidisciplinary treatment planning	161	CGA influenced treatment decisions in 82% of the studied older cancer patients.	Chaibi, 2010[14]
Academic hospital	France	Referral to geriatrician/ multidisciplinary treatment planning	375	20.8% of patients had a change in treatment plan, main factors associated with change: ADL impairment, malnutrition.	Caillet, 2011[28]
Academic hospital	France	Cohort observational study: referral to an oncogeriatric unit prior to or during oncologic treatment	65	Weight loss = main feature prompting patient referral. Patients referred prior to chemotherapy for CGA were more likely to receive adjusted therapy.	Lazarovici, 2011[39]

Abbreviations: HCC, hepatocellular carcinoma; OS, overall survival; QOL, quality of life.

Prospective Cohort Studies

A pilot study in older patients after surgery for early breast cancer demonstrated that 6 months of repeated geriatric assessment generated an average of 17 interventions per patient.[27] Of these interventions, 26% were multidisciplinary and 14% involved the nurse practitioner, 16% the social worker, 17% the dietitian, and 27% the pharmacist. In all, 87% of the interventions were deemed successful, with a decrease of indicators such as inadequate medications or unmet community needs. The mean Functional Assessment of Cancer Treatment–Breast score also improved during the study.

Chaibi and colleagues[14] conducted a prospective study investigating the influence of geriatric consultation with CGA on final therapeutic decision in 161 elderly cancer patients. According to the oncologists' prior decisions after oncogeriatric multidisciplinary consultation, there were no changes in treatment decisions in only 29 patients. Cancer treatment was changed in 79 patients (49%) including delayed therapy in 5 patients, less intensive therapy in 29 patients, and more intensive therapy in 45 patients. Patients for whom the final decision was delayed or who underwent less intensive therapy had significantly more frequent severe comorbidities (23/34, $P<.01$) and dependence for at least one ADL (19/34, $P<.01$). In this study, comprehensive geriatric evaluation did significantly influence treatment decisions in 82% of the studied older cancer patients. In contrast, a later study[15] reported less impact of CGA in the final treatment decision. Of the 30 patients who underwent CGA, in 6 patients the treatment plan was undecided at time of referral. In 5 of these (83%), CGA impacted the ultimate decision. Where the management plan was decided at time of referral (n = 24), CGA impacted the final decision in only 1 patient (4%). Therefore, the impact of CGA in informing treatment decisions was modest but may be of value when the initial treatment decision is uncertain.

The ELCAPA study prospectively followed patients with solid tumors in a large teaching hospital.[28] A total of 656 patients were diagnosed with cancer and had an a priori treatment plan defined. Of these, 392 were referred to a geriatrician and 375 were discussed at a multidisciplinary meeting in which the final cancer treatment plan was decided. A change from the initial treatment plan was made in 20.8% of patients. Intensification of treatment was offered to 10.2% of patients, delay to allow geriatric management was offered to 9%, and decrease in treatment intensity was offered to 80.8%. The prevalence of geriatric problems was high. The median number of altered geriatric parameters was 3 in the group without change and 5 in the group with changes. In multivariate analysis, the parameters associated with changes in treatment were functional impairment (odds ratio [OR] per 0.5 decrease in ADL score: 1.25), and malnutrition (OR 2.99). Trends were also observed for depression and the number of comorbidities. Changes in the global patient management were also recommended by the geriatrician: change in medications in 30.7% of patients, social support in 41.9%, physical therapy in 41.9%, nutritional care in 69.9%, psychological care in 35.7%, memory evaluation in 20.8%, and investigations in 54.9%. The investigators did not assess what prompted patient referrals to the geriatrician. In a smaller study of 65 patients, another group noted that patients referred to a geriatric oncology unit prior to oncologic treatment were more likely to have had recent weight loss than those referred during treatment (32.3% vs 15.3%, P = .03).[39]

Girre and colleagues[20] analyzed 105 patients who had been referred to a geriatric oncology clinic. After the multidisciplinary evaluation, the original treatment plan was modified in 38.7% of patients. These modifications mostly affected patients who planned to receive a treatment involving chemotherapy, and the main modifications were either choosing alternative regimens or another treatment strategy.

FEASIBILITY OF CGA

The feasibility of CGA is an important factor for its implementation in clinical trials. This concept was examined in a questionnaire study[7] in which 245 of 250 patients completed the CGA questionnaire. Most patients (78%) completed the questionnaire on their own and reported acceptance of questionnaire length (91%), no difficult questions (94%), no upsetting questions (96%), and no missing questions (89%). The mean time to completion was 15 minutes, with a median of 12.5 (SD 10, range 2–60). The Cancer and Leukemia Group B study[16] evaluated the implementation of CGA in the cooperative group setting and showed similar results. Of the 85 assessable patients in this trial, the median time to complete the geriatric assessment tool was 22 minutes; 87% of patients (n = 74) completed their portion without assistance, 92% (n = 78) were satisfied with the questionnaire length, and 95% (n = 81) reported no difficult questions. The investigators concluded that the self-administered geriatric assessment tool met the protocol-specified criteria for inclusion in future cooperative group clinical trials.

SUMMARY

The sum of these intervention studies suggests that a CGA can be performed in a variety of settings (inpatient, outpatient, or home), is a multidisciplinary effort, and can lead to interventions that may decrease the risk of morbidity and mortality in older patients with cancer. Further studies are needed using a CGA to (1) guide and test interventions to improve the care of older adults with cancer and (2) evaluate the impact of cancer therapy on geriatric assessment domains.

REFERENCES

1. Barthelemy P, Heitz D, Mathelin C, et al. Adjuvant chemotherapy in elderly patients with early breast cancer. Impact of age and comprehensive geriatric assessment on tumor board proposals. Crit Rev Oncol Hematol 2010;79:196–204.
2. Cudennec T, Gendry T, Labrune S, et al. Use of a simplified geriatric evaluation in thoracic oncology. Lung Cancer 2010;67:232–6.
3. Pilotto A, Ferrucci L, Franceschi M, et al. Development and validation of a multidimensional prognostic index for one-year mortality from comprehensive geriatric assessment in hospitalized older patients. Rejuvenation Res 2008;11:151–61.
4. Wedding U, Kodding D, Pientka L, et al. Physicians' judgement and comprehensive geriatric assessment (CGA) select different patients as fit for chemotherapy. Crit Rev Oncol Hematol 2007;64:1–9.
5. Tulner LR, van Campen JP, Frankfort SV, et al. Changes in under-treatment after comprehensive geriatric assessment: an observational study. Drugs Aging 2010;27:831–43.
6. Kim YJ, Kim JH, Park MS, et al. Comprehensive geriatric assessment in Korean elderly cancer patients receiving chemotherapy. J Cancer Res Clin Oncol 2010;137:839–47.
7. Hurria A, Lichtman SM, Gardes J, et al. Identifying vulnerable older adults with cancer: integrating geriatric assessment into oncology practice. J Am Geriatr Soc 2007;55:1604–8.
8. Winkelmann N, Petersen I, Kiehntopf M, et al. Results of comprehensive geriatric assessment effect survival in patients with malignant lymphoma. J Cancer Res Clin Oncol 2011;137:733–8.

9. Arnoldi E, Dieli M, Mangia M, et al. Comprehensive geriatric assessment in elderly cancer patients: an experience in an outpatient population. Tumori 2007;93:23–5.

10. Clough-Gorr KM, Stuck AE, Thwin SS, et al. Older breast cancer survivors: geriatric assessment domains are associated with poor tolerance of treatment adverse effects and predict mortality over 7 years of follow-up. J Clin Oncol 2010;28:380–6.

11. Pope D, Ramesh H, Gennari R, et al. Pre-operative assessment of cancer in the elderly (PACE): a comprehensive assessment of underlying characteristics of elderly cancer patients prior to elective surgery. Surg Oncol 2006;15:189–97.

12. Kristjansson SR, Nesbakken A, Jordhoy MS, et al. Comprehensive geriatric assessment can predict complications in elderly patients after elective surgery for colorectal cancer: a prospective observational cohort study. Crit Rev Oncol Hematol 2010;76: 208–17.

13. Tucci A, Ferrari S, Bottelli C, et al. A comprehensive geriatric assessment is more effective than clinical judgment to identify elderly diffuse large cell lymphoma patients who benefit from aggressive therapy. Cancer 2009;115:4547–53.

14. Chaibi P, Magne N, Breton S, et al. Influence of geriatric consultation with comprehensive geriatric assessment on final therapeutic decision in elderly cancer patients. Crit Rev Oncol Hematol 2010;79:302–7.

15. Horgan AM, Leighl NB, Coate L, et al. Impact and feasibility of a comprehensive geriatric assessment in the oncology setting: a pilot study. Am J Clin Oncol 2011. [Epub ahead of print].

16. Hurria A, Cirrincione CT, Muss HB, et al. Implementing a geriatric assessment in cooperative group clinical cancer trials: CALGB 360401. J Clin Oncol 2011;29: 1290–6.

17. Extermann M. Basic assessment of the older cancer patient. Curr Treat Options Oncol 2011;12:276–85.

18. Extermann M, Overcash J, Lyman GH, et al. Comorbidity and functional status are independent in older cancer patients. J Clin Oncol 1998;16:1582–7.

19. Ingram SS, Seo PH, Martell RE, et al. Comprehensive assessment of the elderly cancer patient: the feasibility of self-report methodology. J Clin Oncol 2002;20: 770–5.

20. Girre V, Falcou MC, Gisselbrecht M, et al. Does a geriatric oncology consultation modify the cancer treatment plan for elderly patients? J Gerontol A Biol Sci Med Sci 2008;63:724–30.

21. Repetto L, Fratino L, Audisio RA, et al. Comprehensive geriatric assessment adds information to Eastern Cooperative Oncology Group performance status in elderly cancer patients: an Italian Group for Geriatric Oncology Study. J Clin Oncol 2002;20: 494–502.

22. Koroukian SM, Murray P, Madigan E. Comorbidity, disability, and geriatric syndromes in elderly cancer patients receiving home health care. J Clin Oncol 2006;24:2304–10.

23. Maione P, Perrone F, Gallo C, et al. Pretreatment quality of life and functional status assessment significantly predict survival of elderly patients with advanced non-small-cell lung cancer receiving chemotherapy: a prognostic analysis of the multicenter Italian lung cancer in the elderly study. J Clin Oncol 2005;23:6865–72.

24. Retornaz F, Seux V, Sourial N, et al. Comparison of the health and functional status between older inpatients with and without cancer admitted to a geriatric/internal medicine unit. J Gerontol A Biol Sci Med Sci 2007;62:917–22.

25. Flood KL, Carroll MB, Le CV, et al. Geriatric syndromes in elderly patients admitted to an oncology-acute care for elders unit. J Clin Oncol 2006;24:2298–303.

26. Puts MT, Monette J, Girre V, et al. Are frailty markers useful for predicting treatment toxicity and mortality in older newly diagnosed cancer patients? Results from a prospective pilot study. Crit Rev Oncol Hematol 2011;78:138–49.
27. Extermann M, Meyer J, McGinnis M, et al. A comprehensive geriatric intervention detects multiple problems in older breast cancer patients. Crit Rev Oncol Hematol 2004;49:69–75.
28. Caillet P, Canoui-Poitrine F, Vouriot J, et al. Comprehensive geriatric assessment in the decision-making process in elderly patients with cancer: ELCAPA Study. J Clin Oncol 2011;29:3636–42.
29. Freyer G, Geay JF, Touzet S, et al. Comprehensive geriatric assessment predicts tolerance to chemotherapy and survival in elderly patients with advanced ovarian carcinoma: a GINECO study. Ann Oncol 2005;16:1795–800.
30. Audisio RA, Ramesh H, Longo WE, et al. Preoperative assessment of surgical risk in oncogeriatric patients. Oncologist 2005;10:262–8.
31. Extermann M, Boler I, Reich RR, et al. Predicting the risk of chemotherapy toxicity in older patients: The Chemotherapy Risk Assessment Scale for High-Age Patients (CRASH) Score. Cancer 2011. [Epub ahead of print].
32. Basso U, Falci C, Brunello A, et al. Prognostic value of multidimensional geriatric assessment (MGA) on survival of a prospective cohort of 880 elderly cancer patients (ECP) [abstract]. J Clin Oncol 2011;29(Suppl):9065.
33. Hurria A, Togawa K, Mohile SG, et al. Predicting chemotherapy toxicity in older adults with cancer: a prospective multicenter study. J Clin Oncol 2011;29:3457–65.
34. Kanesvaran R, Li H, Koo KN, et al. Analysis of prognostic factors of comprehensive geriatric assessment and development of a clinical scoring system in elderly Asian patients with cancer. J Clin Oncol 2011;29:3620–7.
35. McCorkle R, Strumpf NE, Nuamah IF, et al. A specialized home care intervention improves survival among older post-surgical cancer patients. J Am Geriatr Soc 2000;48:1707–13.
36. Goodwin JS, Satish S, Anderson ET, et al. Effect of nurse case management on the treatment of older women with breast cancer. J Am Geriatr Soc 2003;51:1252–9.
37. Rao AV, Hsieh F, Feussner JR, et al. Geriatric evaluation and management units in the care of the frail elderly cancer patient. J Gerontol A Biol Sci Med Sci 2005;60:798–803.
38. Soejono C. The role of comprehensive geriatric assessment (CGA) in the management of stage 3 hepatocellular carcinoma in the elderly. Crit Rev Oncol Hematol 2006;60:S20.
39. Lazarovici C, Khodabakhshi R, Leignel P, et al. Factors leading oncologists to refer elderly cancer patients for geriatric assessment. J Geriatr Oncol 2011;2:194–9.
40. Bouchardy C, Rapiti E, Fioretta G, et al. Undertreatment strongly decreases prognosis of breast cancer in elderly women. J Clin Oncol 2003;21:3580–7.

Management of Cancer in the Older Adult

Deepak Kilari, MD, Supriya Gupta Mohile, MD, MS*

KEYWORDS

- Elderly • Cancer management • Biology of cancer
- Physiologic changes in the elderly, management

Cancer is primarily a disease of the elderly. According to the National Cancer Institute's Surveillance Epidemiology and End Results (SEER) data, between the years 2003 and 2008 the median age at diagnosis for cancer of all sites was 66 years of age, with 54% of all cancers and 69.5% of all cancer deaths occurring in patients aged 65 years or older. With a steady increase in the average life expectancy and with the recent transition of the Baby Boomers into the over-65 age group, there has been a rapid rise in the elderly population. These statistics portend a growing number of older persons who will succumb to various cancers.

At present sufficient data are lacking regarding the optimal management of cancer in the older population due to underrepresentation of this population in clinical trials.[1,2] Overall the number of persons aged 70 and over who have participated in the clinical trials that have established the evidence base for our treatments is low.[3] Oncology clinical trials also have traditionally excluded patients with comorbidity or disability, which further reduces the generalization of results. In addition, the end points of most cancer clinical trials do not address the maintenance of functional status and quality of life, which may be of more importance to this population than survival.[4] Elderly patients have unique health concerns that can impact cancer care, such as comorbidities, functional and/or cognitive impairment, and lack of social and/or financial support. A comprehensive geriatric assessment (CGA) has promise for guiding oncologists in the management of older patients with cancer.

In this article the authors provide a review of the existing literature regarding the management of common advanced cancers in the elderly.

BIOLOGY OF CANCER IN THE ELDERLY

Aging and cancer are closely interwoven. The incidence of malignant tumors progressively increases with aging in both animals and humans[5] and similarly with

---

Conflict of interest: Dr Kilari: none, Dr Mohile: none.

Department of Medicine, Hematology/Oncology, James P. Wilmot Cancer Center, University of Rochester, 601 Elmwood Avenue, Box 704, Rochester, NY, 14642, USA

* Corresponding author.

E-mail address: supriya_mohile@urmc.rochester.edu

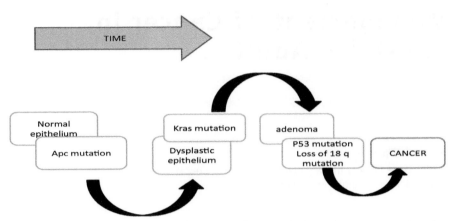

Fig. 1. A genetic model for colorectal cancer carcinogenesis. Apc, adenomatous polyposis

carcinogenesis, there is acceleration of aging processes.[6] Progeroid syndromes that are associated with accelerated aging such as Bloom syndrome, Werner syndrome, and Rothmund-Thomson syndrome are also associated with cancer.[7] For example, Werner syndrome, a rare autosomal disorder, has been linked to a gene belonging to RecQ helicase family essential for DNA homeostasis and has a predisposition to malignancies, mainly sarcomas, in the 30 to 40 age group.[8]

Several mechanisms have been postulated to explain the association between aging and cancer. Genomic instability is a hallmark of both aging and carcinogenesis. Endogenous oxygen radicals, exogenous stresses, and defective DNA repair lead to genomic instability and act synergistically to promote the development of cancer. Colon cancer, which occurs via an intermediate precursor—the adenomatous polyp—represents an ideal model for the multistep genetic changes required over time for cancer development.[9,10] Mutations in tumor suppressor genes such as inactivation of the APC and DCC genes and subsequent additional genetic defects in oncogenes such as K-Ras as depicted in **Fig. 1** represent this stepwise accumulation. Li-Fraumeni syndromes, the familial forms of breast and ovarian cancers, as well as ataxia telangiectasia are consequences of genomic instability in the p53, BRCA, and ATM kinase genes, respectively.[11]

Age-related progressive changes in the immune and endocrine systems help to provide an environment that facilitates cancer development. Observational studies have noted that transformed rat hepatocytic cell lines were only weakly tumorigenic in transplanted young rats compared with older recipients,[12] suggesting the importance of microenvironment. Cells with mismatch repair defects accumulate base mispairing leading to microsatellite instability and leaving the cell vulnerable to uncontrolled cell growth, as demonstrated in hereditary nonpolyposis colon cancer and sporadic colon cancer.[13]

Telomere dysfunction and increased epigenetic gene silencing have also been implicated in the pathogenesis of cancers. Telomeres are essential for chromosomal stability. With aging there is a progressive shortening in their length, which interferes with cell division. This instability at the cellular level increases the rate of somatic mutations that predispose to cancer and other disorders like aplastic anemia. Paradoxically, human cancers have developed mechanisms to maintain telomere length for survival. Autophagy is interrupted with aging, which leads to the accumulation of damaged proteins and mitochondria, which in turn is a source for reactive oxygen species that can contribute to cancer.

DECISION-MAKING FOR TREATMENT IN THE OLDER CANCER PATIENT

Oncologists are often faced with the challenge of making management decisions in the elderly in the absence of evidence-based guidelines.[14] Aging is associated with a multitude of physiologic changes, which in turn are magnified by medical comorbidities and other geriatric problems.[15] Because of these physiologic changes in the elderly, there is potential for an increase in adverse events associated with standard chemotherapy and other cancer management options. However, there is no absolute resistance to chemotherapy based on age. Appropriate treatment for cancer can be safe and effective in the elderly if an adequate assessment is done and appropriate precautions are undertaken. Unfortunately, the fear of treatment-related adverse effects and lack of evidence-based data lead to the undertreatment of cancer in this population.[16] Life expectancy based on chronologic age is heterogeneous. Comorbidities, disability, and geriatric syndromes have a substantial impact on life expectancy. After estimating life expectancy, it should be determined whether the suggested treatment benefit will likely occur in the remaining life span. This consideration is especially important when making treatment decisions about adjuvant therapy. In the absence of a survival gain, quality of life issues should be considered in choosing treatment options.

In the next section the authors discuss the changes associated with aging and the role of a CGA in assisting with treatment decisions.

PHYSIOLOGIC CHANGES WITH AGING

Understanding the physiologic aspects of aging is important, because these changes have implications for efficacy and tolerance of chemotherapy. With aging there are anatomic and structural changes that can adversely impact physiologic reserve in all organ systems. Cancer treatment should be tailored to minimize toxicity, because the loss of reserve is variable. There are several changes that are important to consider. Older patients have decreased cardiac reserve. Both conventional chemotherapies like doxorubicin and targeted agents like alemtuzumab[17] can potentiate heart failure and arrhythmia. The elderly are at increased susceptibility for mucositis secondary to change in the mucosal protective mechanism.[18]

Intestinal motility, absorptive surface area, and gastrointestinal (GI) blood flow are also decreased, which may increase GI toxicity.[19] A decrease in the vital capacity of the lungs in the elderly along with impaired gas exchange can increase the toxicity of radiation.[20] Diminished glomerular filtration rate in the elderly leads to an increased half-life of many drugs and may necessitate dose reduction. The older population is especially at increased susceptibly to confusion, syncope, and falls because of impairment of change in arterial pressure, cerebral blood flow, and disequilibrium. The time to recovery from damage is also prolonged and is particularly relevant to tissues such as the bone marrow and heart muscle. Dysregulated bone marrow can increase the risk of infection, anemia, and thrombocytopenia, with adverse impact on prognosis.[21] Age-related changes in physiology along with their impact on cancer management and suggested interventions are described in **Table 1**.

COMPREHENSIVE GERIATRIC ASSESSMENT

Few oncology trials that have provided evidence for cancer treatment in the elderly have included CGA.[22] CGA is a tool to assess the global health of an older patient and

Table 1
Physiologic changes with aging and suggested interventions

System	Changes	Intervention
Cardiovascular	• Increased risk of drug-related cardiomyopathy • Increased risk of arrhythmia • Increased risk of orthostatic hypotension • Decreased cardiac reserve	• Use liposomal formation of doxorubicin when available • Use cardioprotective-like dexrazoxane • Assess ejection fraction prior to the start of cardiotoxic drugs
GI	• Increased risk of aspiration • Increased susceptibility to mucositis • Decrease in motility and pancreatic exocrine function • Decrease in the admission of hepatic eliminated drugs	• Aggressive oral care • Appropriate bowel regimen, especially with opiates • Avoid concurrent drugs that are metabolized through cytochrome P450 enzyme system
Pulmonary	• Decrease in the pulmonary capacity and reserve • Increased risk of pulmonary infections	• Assessment of influenza and pneumococcal vaccine status • Smoking cessation • Frequent spirometry measurement of pulmonary reserve while on radiotherapy
Renal	• Decrease in the glomerular filtration rate • Increase risk of electrolyte abnormality and calcium • Changes in the efficacy and side effect of the lipid and water-soluble drugs due to change in the distribution	• Dose adjustment of renal excreted drugs • Adequate hydration • Intravenous fluids and urinary alkalinization when administering methotrexate • Monitoring serum electrolytes during therapy • Avoid concurrent nephrotoxic drugs
Immunologic	• Increased susceptibility to infections • Altered T cell function may lead to alteration in stem cell engraftment • Increased risk of cancer due to altered immune surveillance	• Instituting early and appropriate antibiotic treatment • Being aware of the potential risk of infections
Hematologic	• Decreased bone marrow reserve • Increased risk of developing anemia • Increased risk of developing thrombocytopenia • Increased risk of febrile neutropenia	• Maintain hemoglobin • Administer colony-stimulating factors as a primary prophylaxis • Diagnosis febrile neutropenia early and provide effective antibiotics

includes an evaluation of the functional status, comorbid medical conditions, cognition, nutrition, polypharmacy, psychological status, social support, and geriatric syndromes. Each domain is an independent predictor of morbidity and mortality in the older patient.[23–25] The CGA can detect issues pertinent to cancer management that would go unrecognized otherwise.[26] CGA requires a multidisciplinary approach and analysis of the data to create a personalized plan. Incorporation of a CGA into care of elder patients has been shown to improve outcomes by preventing disability and

> **Box 1**
> **Stages of aging using the CGA**
>
> FIT (excellent, good)
> - No functional impairment
> - No significant comorbidities
> - No geriatric syndromes
>
> Vulnerable (good, fair)
> - Dependence in an instrumental activity of daily living but not activities of daily living
> - Comorbidities but not severe or life threatening
> - No geriatric syndromes other than mild memory disorder or mild depression
>
> Frail (poor)
> - Dependence in activities of daily living
> - 3 or more comorbidities or one life-threatening
> - A clinically significant geriatric syndrome

reducing hospitalizations. Recent studies have shown that CGA is feasible in oncology clinical assessment and in cooperative group clinical trials and that factors within CGA can predict toxicity.[27]

Nearly 85% of prostate cancer (CaP) patients and a majority of elderly patients with other cancers have geriatric issues.[28] CGA can help risk-stratify patients into three categories: fit, vulnerable, and frail (**Box 1**). Based on the information derived from the CGA, management options vary (**Fig. 2**). These assessments potentially have the capacity to avoid both over- and undertreatment of cancer in older patients.

In the next sections the authors briefly review the management of prevalent solid tumors in the elderly. The authors focus their review on the management of advanced cancer in the elderly. **Tables 2** and **3** summarize common agents in the treatment of cancer and side effects.

LUNG CANCER

Lung cancer is the leading cause of cancer-related death in Western countries.[29] Management options for lung cancer are based on the cell type. Non–small cell cancer constitutes around 80% of all lung cancers, whereas small cell makes up the remaining. The majority of patients with lung cancer present with stage 4 disease, with which the goal of therapy is palliative.

Non–Small Cell Cancers

In developed countries, the median age at diagnosis of non–small cancer is 68 years, and up to 40% of the patients are older than 70 years at diagnosis.[30] The survival rate decreases with increasing age.[31] The efficacy and tolerability of the standard cisplatin-based regimens is a concern for the elderly population.[32] Cisplatin is associated with both hematologic and nonhematologic toxicity (severe and delayed nausea, emesis, neurotoxicity, ototoxicity, and nephrotoxicity). A metaanalysis of 52 trials comparing chemotherapy with best supportive care, however, indicated that chemotherapy is not associated with a worse outcome in

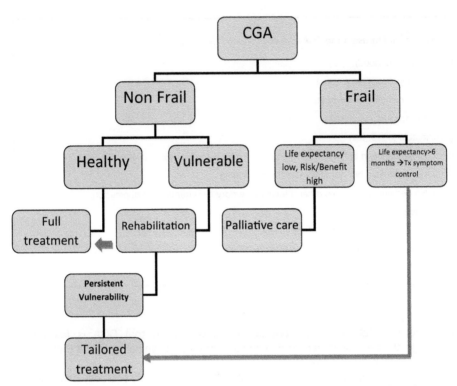

Fig. 2. Stratification of patients based on CGA and suggested treatment algorithm. Tx, treatment.

the elderly and thus paved the way for exploration of better suited regimens.[33] The Elderly lung Cancer Vinorelbine Italian Study trial, which compared single agent vinorelbine to best supportive care in the elderly, showed an improvement not only in overall survival but also in quality of life. Given the conflicting results of the role of combination therapy, single agent is preferred for vulnerable older patients.

Combination chemotherapy with a platinum doublet continues to remain the standard of care for patients in the "young-old" age category who are fit. Retrospective analysis of large randomized controlled trials that have looked into the role of platinum-based chemotherapy for elderly patients noted a similar survival benefit as in the young, with a predictable increase in toxicity.[34] Results from these trials, however, cannot be extrapolated to the general elderly population because they are potentially biased by selection criteria that govern enrollment. The results of the French Intergroup trial (IFCT-0501), the only trial to assess the efficacy of a platinum doublet in the elderly in a prospective manner, demonstrated an overall survival benefit.[35]

The safety profile and ease of administration of targeted therapy makes these agents suitable alternative therapies for the elderly. Erlotinib, an epidermal growth factor receptor (EGFR) inhibitor, has shown a survival benefit in patients for whom both first and second line treatments have failed[36] and is being tested in the first line setting. Rash and diarrhea are the most common reported toxicities on this regimen, and these side effects could be of greater consequence in the elderly.

Table 2
Common side effects of commonly used chemotherapeutic agents

Drugs	Cancers Used In	Side Effects
Cisplatin (alkylating agent)	Gastric/esophagus Bladder Lung	Emesis Neurotoxicity Nephrotoxicity Ototoxicity
Docetaxel (binds microtubules)	Prostate Breast Bladder Esophagus	Fluid retention Myelosuppression Neurosensory events Emesis
Oxaliplatin (alkylating agent)	Pancreas Gastric/esophagus Colon	Fatigue Myelosuppression Peripheral neuropathy Emesis
Capecitabine (antimetabolite)	Colon Breast Pancreas Gastric/esophagus	Hand-foot syndrome Myelosuppression Diarrhea Elevated Liver function tests
Gemcitabine (pyrimidine antimetabolite)	Pancreas Lung Breast Bladder	Flulike symptoms Rash Myelosuppression GI side effects
5-Fluorouracil (antimetabolite)	Pancreas Colon Gastric/esophagus	Cardiovascular (arrhythmia, vasospasm, heart failure, ventricular ectopy) Dermatologic (alopecia, dermatitis etc) Myelosuppression

Small Cell Lung Cancer

Small cell lung cancer (SCLC) represents a significant problem in the elderly, with around 32% of all newly diagnosed cases detected in patients older than 70 years of age and 10% detected in octogenarians.[37] SCLC is characterized by a rapid doubling time and propensity for early metastasis. Small cell is highly responsive to chemotherapy and radiotherapy, but prognosis is still poor given rapid development of resistance. In patients with extensive stage SCLC, a response is seen in 60% to 70% of patients; however, relapse is common, and only 5% of patients with SCLC are alive at 5 years. Because a small percentage of patients can be cured, an aggressive approach is favored when feasible.

Platinum-based combination chemotherapy is the backbone of treatment in patients with extensive stage SCLC. Carboplatin and etoposide is the most investigated regimen and has been shown to have a similar benefit in terms of overall survival with a predictable increase in toxicity when compared with the young.[38] Carboplatin is advantageous in the elderly because of the ease of administration and decreased toxicity and has largely replaced cisplatin the elderly. When considering prophylactic cranial irradiation to reduce the risk of symptomatic brain metastasis in the elderly, the relative benefit as well as neurocognitive changes should be taken into account.

PROSTATE CANCER

CaP affects the elderly disproportionately. The estimated prevalence of CaP in men aged 75 years and older is over 1 million, with over 60% of all the new cases

Table 3
Targeted agents and common side effects

Drugs	Cancer	Side Effects
Bevacizumab (VEGF inhibitors)	Colon Breast Renal	Elevated blood pressure Thromboembolic events Proteinuria Upper respiratory tract infections
Cetuximab (EGFR inhibitor)	Colon Head and neck	Fatigue Acneiform rash GI toxicity
Erlotinib	Pancreas Lung	Rash Fatigue Rash GI toxicity
Sunitinib (VEGF inhibitor)	Renal cell Pancreatic neuroendocrine Thyroid	Hypothyroidism Heart failure Hand-foot syndrome Hypertension Diarrhea Nausea
Everolimus	Renal cell carcinoma Pancreatic neuroendocrine	GI toxicity Hypercholesterolemia Hyperglycemia Rash

Abbreviations: EGFR, epidermal growth factor receptor; VEGF, vascular endothelial growth factor inhibitor.

diagnosed in men older than 65 years.[39] Because of the long natural history of the disease, the case fatality rate is low in the young. However, 70% of men who die of CaP are 75 years and older.

Advanced Prostate Cancer

Advanced CaP cannot be cured and includes disease that has spread outside the prostate and/or is symptomatic, as well as biochemical recurrence only (a rise in prostate-specific antigen with no evidence of disease). Androgen deprivation therapy (ADT) is used in the initial management of these patients and is associated with a multitude of side effects including weakness, physical performance problems, and cognitive/mood disorders. ADT consists of gonadotropin-releasing hormone agonist/ antagonist as well as antiandrogen, and their effect lies in their ability to lower the testosterone levels available to the cancer cells. The use of intermittent ADT to decrease the side effect profile is currently under evaluation. Given the significant adverse effects associated with the use of ADT in older patients, serious consideration must be undertaken with the patient regarding risks versus benefits prior to initiation. For older patients with indolent cancer characteristics and no clinical symptoms, active surveillance should be considered.

In the elderly, when the disease has progressed on ADT (castration-resistant CaP) standard chemotherapy—docetaxel, 75 mg/m^2 every 3 weeks—should be considered based on the CGA. Subset analysis of the index trials has established that men over 75 years of age had response equivalent to a younger population, with a predictable increase in toxicity.[40,41] A lower dose of docetaxel (ie, 30 mg/m^2 on a weekly basis) has been studied in an attempt to address the issue of myelosuppression and other adverse effects seen with standard dose chemotherapy.[42,43] Results from these studies indicate that this schedule has a modest effect on progression-free survival but did not impact overall survival. These studies had a high percentage of dropout rate (30%)[44] compared with the standard dose (8%), likely because of the older and more vulnerable population included.

Several new regimens have been recently approved in treatment of castration-resistant CaP. Abiraterone, which selectively blocks the cytochrome P450 C17 and thereby inhibits androgen biosynthesis, has been shown to improve overall survival in this setting. The trial that led to its approval included patients who were older than 75 years (28% of the study population) and noted a similar benefit.[45] An improved overall survival was also seen when Sipuleucel-T, an autologous active cellular based immunotherapy, was compared with a placebo in a trial in which the median age was 72 years.[46] De Bono and colleagues[47] compared cabazitaxel with mitoxantrone in patients who progressed on first line docetaxel. The median age in this trial was 67 years, with 20% of the study population being older than 75 years, and cabazitaxel irrespective of age improved overall survival.[47]

BLADDER CANCER

Age is an independent risk factor for the development of transitional cell cancer (TCC) of the bladder.[48] The incidence of TCC is 28.6% in patients under 65 years and 71.4% in those older than 65 years.[49] The median age at diagnosis is 69 years for men and 71 years for women, with the peak incidence at 85 years.[50] With advanced age, there is an increased risk of detecting higher stage and higher grade cancers. The treatment is based on whether the disease is muscle invasive and/or metastatic or not.

Clinically Localized Muscle-Invasive Bladder Cancer

Radical cystectomy with pelvic lymph node dissection and urinary diversion remains the standard of care in patients with muscle-invasive bladder cancer.[51] However, most elderly patients never actually undergo this procedure for a multitude of reasons[52] that include high perioperative morbidity of 30% to 60%. The patients who undergo the procedure still often have poor oncologic outcomes because of inadequate pelvic lymph node dissection and inadequate use of chemotherapy in the neoadjuvant or adjuvant setting.[53] Alternate approaches like extensive transurethral resection and radiation therapy with chemotherapy are at best only palliative. Bladder sparing approaches can be considered in patients who are high risk for surgery, but these approaches are associated with worse overall survival and cancer-specific survival.

Metastatic Disease

Cisplatin-based therapy is the most effective regimen for patients with bladder cancer, but it is associated with various toxicities as described earlier. Because of the high prevalence of impaired renal function and other comorbidities in this population, over 40% of the population are ineligible for a cisplatin-based regimen. In patients who are unfit for this therapy, several other regimens have been studied including single agent gemcitabine, paclitaxel, combination regimens of gemcitabine/Taxol[54] and carboplatin,[55] which have all demonstrated modest activity with good tolerance. Hence, when considering therapy for the elderly, overall benefit should be weighed against the risk of toxicity.

RENAL CELL CANCER

The average age at presentation of renal cell cancer (RCC) is 64 years in both sexes.[56] In the 1990s almost 60% of the cases were diagnosed incidentally compared with the 1970s when only 10% of cancers were found by chance.[57] Patients are more likely to be diagnosed with early stage disease in the current decade than in previous years.[58]

The role of cytoreductive nephrectomy to significantly prolong survival, delay time to progression, and enhance the response to systemic biological therapy in patients with advanced RCC is well-established in select fit patients with metastatic RCC. Kader and colleagues[59] analyzed the potential risk and benefits of this procedure in those over 75 years and noted high perioperative mortality (21% vs 1%) compared with the young. In spite of this increased early death, the median survival was similar in both age groups. Because of the high perioperative mortality, until more data are available in the targeted agent era, it is perhaps reasonable to consider systemic therapy with targeted therapies in lieu of up-front nephrectomy.

In contrast to other malignancies, chemotherapy does not have a role in RCC.[60] For a long time, interleukin-2 and interferon were the only available systemic options for management of RCC. The toxicities of these cytokines, however, were an obstacle to treatment in both the young and elderly. Agents targeting tumor angiogenesis (vascular endothelial growth factor inhibitor; VEGF) and intracellular pathways mediating proliferation and growth (mammalian target of rapamycin inhibitor [mTOR]) have demonstrated improved efficacy with favorable toxicity profile in several phase 2 and 3 trials.[61–63] and have largely replaced cytokine treatments. The median age of patients in most of these trials was 62 years, and in all of these studies, over 30% of the study population was above 65 years.

These targeted agents have unique side effects that can adversely impact outcome in the elderly (see **Table 3**). Retrospective subgroup analysis of these trials suggested a similar benefit in all patient age groups, with similar toxicity and a possible greater impact on quality of life.[64] This analysis, however, may not be representative of the elderly general population because of selection bias. In the absence of prospective controlled comparison between different agents, when selecting an agent, the toxicity profile and implications of specific comorbid conditions should be taken into account.

COLORECTAL CANCER

In the Western world, colorectal cancer (CRC) is one of the most common cancers. The median age at diagnosis is 71 years.[65] CRC is the second most common cause of cancer death in the above-70 age group, with approximately 50% of all CRC occurring in this age group. The standard of care in patients with stage 4 disease is systemic chemotherapy with or without targeted therapy and surgical intervention when appropriate for curative intent or symptom management.

Age per se should not be considered a contraindication for surgery. In patients with liver-only metastasis, hepatic resection can offer a chance of long-term survival.[66] In the select elderly, this procedure is safe and feasible, with a similar progression-free survival and overall survival benefit.[67] Unfortunately, elderly patients who underwent this procedure were less likely to receive perioperative chemotherapy and more likely to have limited surgical procedures.[68]

5-fluorouracil (FU) is the backbone of systemic treatment in patients with metastatic CRC. Infusional 5FU is better tolerated compared with bolus regimens because of its favorable toxicity profile and response. Pooled analysis of 22 studies using a 5FU regimen noted similar toxicity, response rates and overall survival in the elderly when compared with the young.[69] There continues to be an active debate regarding the use of combination therapy versus monotherapy in the management of older patients with metastatic colon cancer because of a similar overall survival benefit noted in several trials.[70] The OPTIMOX-1 approach of combination chemotherapy alternating with 5FU monotherapy as maintenance seems to be a reasonable option.[71] Capecitabine, an oral prodrug of 5FU, was tested in the FOCUS2 trial and was noted to have similar efficacy with increased adverse events. The combination of 5FU with irinotecan[72] and oxaliplatin[73] has noted similar response rates, progression-free survival, and overall survival in all age groups.

The BEAT (Bevacizumab Expanded Access trial) and the BRiTE (Bevacizumab Regimens Investigation of Treatment Effects) noted a similar improvement in progression-free survival in the older patients with the use of bevacizumab, a VEGF antibody. When used in addition to standard chemotherapy, improvement was seen in overall survival and progression-free survival in the elderly.[74] The incidence of arterial thromboembolic events increased with age, and caution must be used when prescribing this regimen in the elderly. The use of antiepidermal growth factor receptors antibody (cetuximab) has had mixed efficacy results in subgroup analyses of patients over the age of 65, and further studies are needed.

UPPER GI TRACT CANCERS
Pancreatic Cancer

Pancreatic adenocarcinoma remains one of the most lethal cancers in the Western world, with the incidence and anticipated death almost identical.[75] The median age at diagnosis is 72 years, with over 68% of patients over the age of 65. Pancreatectomy is potentially curative; however, only 15% to 20% are candidates, because of late presentation.[76] The median survival in patients with advanced disease is 3 to 7 months. Advanced disease refers to unresectable and metastatic disease.

Gemcitabine remains the backbone of chemotherapy in patients with advanced disease, with a clinical and an overall survival benefit. In spite of a minimal objective response, a clinical benefit, which refers to an improvement in pain, performance status, and weight without deterioration of other factors, mainly led to the approval of this drug.[77] Several studies assessed the feasibility of this regimen in the elderly and noted similar tolerance and benefit as in the young.[78-80] The ACCORD trial, which compared FOLFIRINOX (5FU/leucovorin, irinotecan, and oxaliplatin) with gemcitabine noted improvement in overall response rate, progression-free survival, and overall survival with combination chemotherapy at the expense of an increase in toxicity, manly neutropenia.[81] The trial included only patients with good performance status and under 75 years of age, and in view of significant toxicity, is a challenging regimen for the elderly. Various combinations of gemcitabine have been tested with no improvement in outcome except for erlotinib, an EGFR inhibitor that showed a small but statistically significant benefit but with increased toxicity.[82] In the absence of better data, gemcitabine alone is a safe option in select elderly.

Gastric/Esophageal Cancer

Cancers originating in the lower esophagus, gastroesophageal junction, and gastric area are treated similarly because they share common pathogenesis, regardless of histology. Approximately 61% and 64% of esophageal and gastric cancers arise in patients over 65 years of age. Fit elderly patients with resectable disease should be considered for perioperative chemotherapy.[83]

In the elderly with recurrent and metastatic disease, palliative chemotherapy not only improves overall survival but also quality of life. The efficacy and tolerability of platinum-containing regimen in this population was established by Trumper and colleagues.[84] In a pooled analyses of three trials, the investigators were able to demonstrate an equivalent benefit of chemotherapy in the elderly (>70 years) as in the young. The REAL study[85] and phase 3, V325 Belgian trial[86] noted that platinum-based three-drug regimens resulted in prolonged median time to progression with a clinical benefit and could be tolerated in select elderly.

The major drawback to these regimens was the need for a central venous line for administration and high incidence of line-related complications. The REAL-2 trial noted similar outcomes when capecitabine was substituted for infusional 5FU, and when oxaliplatin was substituted for cisplatin.[87] Because of ease of administration with better side effect profile, this regimen should be considered. In the elderly who cannot tolerate combination chemotherapy, single agent 5FU or capecitabine are reasonable options.

SUPPORTIVE CARE

Nausea and vomiting remain the most feared complications of cancer treatment (surgery, radiation, chemotherapy, or a combination). The intrinsic emetogenic nature of each type of chemotherapy is well-established, and treatment is recommended based on the risk. Corticosteroids, 5 Ht3 antagonists, and aprepitant are commonly used, both as monotherapy and in combination in the young and elderly alike, with good response. Morbidity related to skeletal events is common in cancer patients due to metastasis to bone and cancer treatment–induced bone loss. Bisphosphonates and other osteoclast inhibitors like denosumab are effective mainly by decreasing skeletal-related events. All these patients are also advised to receive supplemental calcium and vitamin D. Renal insufficiency and osteonecrosis of the jaw can occur rarely as side effects with treatment. Chronic pain is common in elderly patients with cancer. Management requires ongoing assessment and recognition of age-related changes. Medications with a short half-life and small doses are better tolerated. When prescribing opiates, additive effect should be taken into account.

SUMMARY

Cancer incidence and mortality rise exponentially in the elderly. With the aging of the population there is an urgent need to address this issue with evidence-based guidelines. Delayed diagnosis and incomplete workup and treatment are well-documented in this population. Incorporation of a geriatric evaluation in oncology practice should be routinely implemented to prevent adverse outcomes. Treatment decisions in the elderly should not be based solely on survival gains but should also take quality of life into consideration. Cancer treatment is safe and effective in the elderly population. Social issues and other comorbidities should be addressed to improve compliance and outcome. Many unanswered questions regarding the optimal management of elderly cancer patients can be addressed only with the new clinical trials. Eliminating age bias among health care providers by providing education will help achieve optimal care for the elderly with cancer.

REFERENCES

1. Hutchins LF, Unger JM, Crowley JJ, et al. Underrepresentation of patients 65 years of age or older in cancer-treatment trials. N Engl J Med 1999;341(27):2061–7.

2. Lang KJ, Lidder S. Under-representation of the elderly in cancer clinical trials. Br J Hosp Med (Lond) 2010;71(12):678–81.
3. Trimble EL, Carter CL, Cain D, et al. Representation of older patients in cancer treatment trials. Cancer 1994;74(7 Suppl):2208–14.
4. Husain LS, Collins K, Reed M, et al. Choices in cancer treatment: a qualitative study of the older women's (>70 years) perspective. Psychooncology 2008;17(4):410–6.
5. Dix D, Cohen P. On the role of aging in carcinogenesis. Anticancer Res 1999;19(1B): 723–6.
6. Teramoto S, Fukuchi Y, Uejima Y, et al. Influences of chronic tobacco smoke inhalation on aging and oxidant-antioxidant balance in the senescence-accelerated mouse (SAM)-P/2. Exp Gerontol 1993;28(1):87–95.
7. Bohr VA. Human premature aging syndromes and genomic instability. Mech Ageing Dev 2002;123(8):987–93.
8. Epstein CJ, Martin GM, Schultz AL, et al. Werner's syndrome a review of its symptomatology, natural history, pathologic features, genetics and relationship to the natural aging process. Medicine (Baltimore) 1966;45(3):177–221.
9. Fearon ER, Vogelstein B. A genetic model for colorectal tumorigenesis. Cell 1990; 61(5):759–67.
10. Ionov Y, Peinado MA, Malkhosyan S, et al. Ubiquitous somatic mutations in simple repeated sequences reveal a new mechanism for colonic carcinogenesis. Nature 1993;363(6429):558–61.
11. Matheu A, Maraver A, Klatt P, et al. Delayed ageing through damage protection by the Arf/p53 pathway. Nature 2007;448(7151):375–9.
12. McCullough KD, Coleman WB, Smith GJ, et al. Age-dependent regulation of the tumorigenic potential of neoplastically transformed rat liver epithelial cells by the liver microenvironment. Cancer Res 1994;54(14):3668–71.
13. Markowitz S, Wang J, Myeroff L, et al. Inactivation of the type II TGF-beta receptor in colon cancer cells with microsatellite instability. Science 1995;268(5215):1336–8.
14. Boyd CM, Darer J, Boult C, et al. Clinical practice guidelines and quality of care for older patients with multiple comorbid diseases: implications for pay for performance. JAMA 2005;294(6):716–24.
15. Koroukian SM, Murray P, Madigan E, et al. Comorbidity, disability, and geriatric syndromes in elderly cancer patients receiving home health care. J Clin Oncol 2006;24(15):2304–10.
16. Bouchardy C, Rapiti E, Fioretta G, et al. Undertreatment strongly decreases prognosis of breast cancer in elderly women. J Clin Oncol Oct 1 2003;21(19):3580–7.
17. Lenihan DJ, Alencar AJ, Yang D, et al. Cardiac toxicity of alemtuzumab in patients with mycosis fungoides/Sezary syndrome. Blood 2004;104(3):655–8.
18. Balducci L, Extermann M. Management of cancer in the older person: a practical approach. Oncologist 2000;5(3):224–37.
19. McLean AJ, Le Couteur DG. Aging biology and geriatric clinical pharmacology. Pharmacol Rev 2004;56(2):163–84.
20. Girinsky T, Cosset JM. [Pulmonary and cardiac late effects of ionizing radiations alone or combined with chemotherapy]. Cancer Radiother 1997;1(6):735–43 [in French].
21. Dees EC, O'Reilly S, Goodman SN, et al. A prospective pharmacologic evaluation of age-related toxicity of adjuvant chemotherapy in women with breast cancer. Cancer Invest 2000;18(6):521–9.
22. Brunello A, Sandri R, Extermann M. Multidimensional geriatric evaluation for older cancer patients as a clinical and research tool. Cancer Treat Rev 2009;35(6):487–92.

23. Reuben DB, Rubenstein LV, Hirsch SH, et al. Value of functional status as a predictor of mortality: results of a prospective study. Am J Med 1992;93(6):663–9 [erratum in Am J Med 199;94(5):560; Am J Med 1993;94(2):232].

24. Newman AB, Yanez D, Harris T, et al. Weight change in old age and its association with mortality. J Am Geriatr Soc 2001;49(10):1309–18.

25. Seeman TE, Berkman LF, Kohout F, et al. Intercommunity variations in the association between social ties and mortality in the elderly. A comparative analysis of three communities. Ann Epidemiol 1993;3(4):325–35.

26. Extermann M, Meyer J, McGinnis M, et al. A comprehensive geriatric intervention detects multiple problems in older breast cancer patients. Crit Rev Oncol Hematol 2004;49(1):69–75.

27. Hurria A, Togawa K, Mohile SG, et al. Predicting chemotherapy toxicity in older adults with cancer: a prospective multicenter study. J Clin Oncol 2011;29(25):3457–65.

28. Extermann M, Hurria A. Comprehensive geriatric assessment for older patients with cancer. J Clin Oncol 2007;25(14):1824–31.

29. Parkin DM. Global cancer statistics in the year 2000. Lancet Oncol 2001;2(9):533–43.

30. Gridelli C, Maione P, Rossi A, et al. Treatment of advanced non-small-cell lung cancer in the elderly. Lung Cancer 2009;66(3):282–6.

31. Fry WA, Phillips JL, Menck HR. Ten-year survey of lung cancer treatment and survival in hospitals in the United States: a national cancer data base report. Cancer 1999; 86(9):1867–76.

32. Langer CJ, Manola J, Bernardo P, et al. Cisplatin-based therapy for elderly patients with advanced non-small-cell lung cancer: implications of Eastern Cooperative Oncology Group 5592, a randomized trial. J Natl Cancer Inst 2002;94(3):173–81.

33. Anonymous. Chemotherapy in non-small cell lung cancer: a meta-analysis using updated data on individual patients from 52 randomised clinical trials. Non-small Cell Lung Cancer Collaborative Group. BMJ 1995;311(7010):899–909.

34. Lilenbaum RC, Herndon JE 2nd, List MA, et al. Single-agent versus combination chemotherapy in advanced non-small-cell lung cancer: the cancer and leukemia group B (study 9730). J Clin Oncol 2005;23(1):190–6.

35. Quoix E, Zalcman GR, Oster JP, et al. Carboplatin and weekly paclitaxel doublet chemotherapy compared with monotherapy in elderly patients with advanced non-small-cell lung cancer: IFCT-0501 randomised, phase 3 trial. Lancet 2011;378(9796):1079–88.

36. Shepherd FA, Rodrigues Pereira J, Ciuleanu T, et al. Erlotinib in previously treated non-small-cell lung cancer. N Engl J Med 2005;353(2):123–32.

37. Owonikoko TK, Ragin CC, Belani CP, et al. Lung cancer in elderly patients: an analysis of the surveillance, epidemiology, and end results database. J Clin Oncol 2007;25(35):5570–7.

38. Larive S, Bombaron P, Riou R, et al. Carboplatin-etoposide combination in small cell lung cancer patients older than 70 years: a phase II trial. Lung Cancer 2002;35(1):1–7.

39. Horner M, Ries L, Krapcho M. SEER cancer statistics review, 1975–2006. Bethesda (MD): National Cancer Institute; 2009.

40. Anderson J, Van Poppel H, Bellmunt J, et al. Chemotherapy for older patients with prostate cancer. BJU Int 2007;99(2):269–73.

41. Berthold DR, Pond GR, Soban F, et al. Docetaxel plus prednisone or mitoxantrone plus prednisone for advanced prostate cancer: updated survival in the TAX 327 study. J Clin Oncol 2008;26(2):242–5.

42. Beer TM, Berry W, Wersinger EM, et al. Weekly docetaxel in elderly patients with prostate cancer: efficacy and toxicity in patients at least 70 years of age compared with patients younger than 70 years. Clin Prostate Cancer 2003;2(3):167–72.

43. Fossa SD. A randomized phase II trial comparing weekly taxotere plus prednisolone versus prednisolone alone in androgen-independent prostate cancer. Front Radiat Ther Oncol 2008;41:108–16.
44. Italiano A, Ortholan C, Oudard S, et al. Docetaxel-based chemotherapy in elderly patients (age 75 and older) with castration-resistant prostate cancer. Eur Urol 2009;55(6):1368–75.
45. de Bono JS, Logothetis CJ, Molina A, et al. Abiraterone and increased survival in metastatic prostate cancer. N Engl J Med 2011;364(21):1995–2005.
46. Kantoff PW, Higano CS, Shore ND, et al. Sipuleucel-T immunotherapy for castration-resistant prostate cancer. N Engl J Med 2010;363(5):411–22.
47. de Bono JS, Oudard S, Ozguroglu M, et al. Prednisone plus cabazitaxel or mitoxantrone for metastatic castration-resistant prostate cancer progressing after docetaxel treatment: a randomised open-label trial. Lancet 2010;376(9747):1147–54.
48. Messing E. Urothelial tumors of the bladder. In: Campbell MF, Wein AJ, Kavoussi LR, et al, editors. Campbell-Walsh urology. 9th edition. Philadelphia: Saunders Elsevier; 2007. p. 2407–46.
49. Jemal A, Siegel R, Ward E, et al. Cancer statistics, 2008. CA Cancer J Clin 2008; 58(2):71–96.
50. Schultzel M, Saltzstein SL, Downs TM, et al. Late age (85 years or older) peak incidence of bladder cancer. J Urol 2008;179(4):1302–6.
51. Stein JP, Lieskovsky G, Cote R, et al. Radical cystectomy in the treatment of invasive bladder cancer: long-term results in 1,054 patients. J Clin Oncol 2001; 19(3):666–75.
52. Prout GR, Wesley MN, Yancik R, et al. Age and comorbidity impact surgical therapy in older bladder carcinoma patients. Cancer 2005;104(8):1638–47.
53. Resorlu B, Beduk Y, Baltaci S, et al. The prognostic significance of advanced age in patients with bladder cancer treated with radical cystectomy. BJU Int 2009;103(4):480–3.
54. Vaughn DJ, Manola J, Dreicer R, et al. Phase II study of paclitaxel plus carboplatin in patients with advanced carcinoma of the urothelium and renal dysfunction (E2896). Cancer 2002;95(5):1022–7.
55. Linardou H, Aravantinos G, Efstathiou E, et al. Gemcitabine and carboplatin combination as first-line treatment in elderly patients and those unfit for cisplatin-based chemotherapy with advanced bladder carcinoma: Phase II study of the Hellenic Co-operative Oncology Group. Urology 2004;64(3):479–84.
56. Murai M. Editorial comment on: impact of gender in renal cell carcinoma: an analysis of the SEER database. Eur Urol 2008;54(1):140–1.
57. Pantuck AJ, Zisman A, Belldegrun AS. The changing natural history of renal cell carcinoma. J Urol 2001;166(5):1611–23.
58. Nguyen MM, Gill IS, Ellison LM, et al The evolving presentation of renal carcinoma in the United States: trends from the Surveillance, Epidemiology, and End Results program. J Urol 2006;176(6 Pt 1):2397–400 [discussion: 2400].
59. Kader AK, Tamboli P, Luongo T, et al. Cytoreductive nephrectomy in the elderly patient: the M. D. Anderson Cancer Center experience. J Urol 2007;177(3):855–61.
60. Vogelzang NJ. Another step toward the cure of metastatic renal cell carcinoma? J Clin Oncol 2010;28(34):5017–9.
61. Escudier B, Eisen T, Stadler WM, et al. Sorafenib in advanced clear-cell renal-cell carcinoma. N Engl J Med 2007;356(2):125–34.
62. Motzer RJ, Hutson TE, Tomczak P, et al. Sunitinib versus interferon alfa in metastatic renal-cell carcinoma. N Engl J Med 2007;356(2):115–24.
63. Hudes G, Carducci M, Tomczak P, et al. Temsirolimus, interferon alfa, or both for advanced renal-cell carcinoma. N Engl J Med 2007;356(22):2271–81.

64. Rini BI, Jaeger E, Weinberg V, et al. Clinical response to therapy targeted at vascular endothelial growth factor in metastatic renal cell carcinoma: impact of patient characteristics and Von Hippel-Lindau gene status. BJU Int 2006;98(4): 756–62.
65. Kohne CH, Folprecht G, Goldberg RM, et al. Chemotherapy in elderly patients with colorectal cancer. Oncologist 2008;13(4):390–402.
66. Fong Y, Fortner J, Sun RL, et al. Clinical score for predicting recurrence after hepatic resection for metastatic colorectal cancer: analysis of 1001 consecutive cases. Ann Surg 1999;230(3):309–18 [discussion: 318–31].
67. Figueras J, Ramos E, Lopez-Ben S, et al. Surgical treatment of liver metastases from colorectal carcinoma in elderly patients. When is it worthwhile? Clin Transl Oncol 2007;9(6):392–400.
68. Adam R, Frilling A, Elias D, et al. Liver resection of colorectal metastases in elderly patients. Br J Surg 2010;97(3):366–76.
69. Folprecht G, Cunningham D, Ross P, et al. Efficacy of 5-fluorouracil-based chemotherapy in elderly patients with metastatic colorectal cancer: a pooled analysis of clinical trials. Ann Oncol 2004;15(9):1330–8.
70. Koopman M, Antonini NF, Douma J, et al. Sequential versus combination chemotherapy with capecitabine, irinotecan, and oxaliplatin in advanced colorectal cancer (CAIRO): a phase III randomised controlled trial. Lancet 2007;370(9582): 135–42.
71. Figer A, Perez-Staub N, Carola E, et al. FOLFOX in patients aged between 76 and 80 years with metastatic colorectal cancer: an exploratory cohort of the OPTIMOX1 study. Cancer 2007;110(12):2666–71.
72. Chiara S, Nobile MT, Vincenti M, et al. Advanced colorectal cancer in the elderly: results of consecutive trials with 5-fluorouracil-based chemotherapy. Cancer Chemother Pharmacol 1998;42(4):336–40.
73. Goldberg RM, Tabah-Fisch I, Bleiberg H, et al. Pooled analysis of safety and efficacy of oxaliplatin plus fluorouracil/leucovorin administered bimonthly in elderly patients with colorectal cancer. J Clin Oncol 2006;24(25):4085–91 [erratum in J Clin Oncol 2008;26(17):2925–6].
74. Cassidy J, Saltz LB, Giantonio BJ, et al. Effect of bevacizumab in older patients with metastatic colorectal cancer: pooled analysis of four randomized studies. J Cancer Res Clin Oncol 2010;136(5):737–43.
75. Li D, Xie K, Wolff R, et al. Pancreatic cancer. Lancet. 2004;363(9414):1049–57.
76. Cooperman AM. Pancreatic cancer: the bigger picture. Surg Clin North Am 2001; 81(3):557–74.
77. Burris HA 3rd, Moore MJ, Andersen J, et al. Improvements in survival and clinical benefit with gemcitabine as first-line therapy for patients with advanced pancreas cancer: a randomized trial. J Clin Oncol 1997;15(6):2403–13.
78. Locher C, Fabre-Guillevin E, Brunetti F, et al. Fixed-dose rate gemcitabine in elderly patients with advanced pancreatic cancer: an observational study. Crit Rev Oncol Hematol 2008;68(2): 178–82.
79. Marechal R, Demols A, Gay F, et al. Tolerance and efficacy of gemcitabine and gemcitabine-based regimens in elderly patients with advanced pancreatic cancer. Pancreas 2008;36(3): e16–21.
80. Katakura Y, Nakahara K, Kobayashi M, et al. [Gemcitabine therapy for unresectable pancreatic cancer in elderly patients]. Nippon Shokakibyo Gakkai Zasshi 2010;107(3): 396–406 [in Japanese].
81. Conroy T, Desseigne F, Ychou M, et al. FOLFIRINOX versus gemcitabine for metastatic pancreatic cancer. N Engl J Med 2011;364(19):1817–25.

82. Moore MJ, Goldstein D, Hamm J, et al. Erlotinib plus gemcitabine compared with gemcitabine alone in patients with advanced pancreatic cancer: a phase III trial of the National Cancer Institute of Canada Clinical Trials Group. J Clin Oncol 2007;25(15): 1960–6.

83. Cunningham D, Allum WH, Stenning SP, et al. Perioperative chemotherapy versus surgery alone for resectable gastroesophageal cancer. N Engl J Med 2006;355(1): 11–20.

84. Trumper M, Ross PJ, Cunningham D, et al. Efficacy and tolerability of chemotherapy in elderly patients with advanced oesophago-gastric cancer: a pooled analysis of three clinical trials. Eur J Cancer 2006;42(7):827–34.

85. Findlay M, Cunningham D, Norman A, et al. A phase II study in advanced gastro-esophageal cancer using epirubicin and cisplatin in combination with continuous infusion 5-fluorouracil (ECF). Ann Oncol 1994 1994;5(7):609–16.

86. Van Cutsem E, Moiseyenko VM, Tjulandin S, et al. Phase III study of docetaxel and cisplatin plus fluorouracil compared with cisplatin and fluorouracil as first-line therapy for advanced gastric cancer: a report of the V325 Study Group. J Clin Oncol 2006;24(31):4991–7.

87. Cunningham D, Starling N, Rao S, et al. Capecitabine and oxaliplatin for advanced esophagogastric cancer. N Engl J Med 2008;358(1):36–46.

Principles of Surgical Oncology in the Elderly

Andrew P. Zbar, MD (Lond), MBBS[a],*, Aviad Gravitz, MD[a],
Riccardo A. Audisio, MD[b]

KEYWORDS

• Cancer • Chemoprevention • Elderly • Treatment

Almost two thirds of all solid tumors are diagnosed in patients over 65 years of age, where the annual age-adjusted incidence of cancer has shown a slow but steady increase by nearly 15% over the last 30 years to 450 cases per 100,000 of the population.[1] This has been coupled with a relative increase in cancer-related mortality when compared with an annual decline in heart-related death rates in the elderly of about 30% over the same period of time.[2,3] The issues involved here are complex, given the increase in life expectancy and the true increase in cancer incidence with advancing age, where the lifetime probability of development of an invasive cancer is nearly 1 in 2 in males and 1 in 3 in females and where the majority of the risk occurs in patients who are over 60 years of age.[4,5] The issues in cancer management in the elderly are complex and include some estimation by the surgical oncologist concerning a risk assessment of survival limitation by the cancer of preexistent, age-related illnesses and a determination of their effect on the delivery of optimal cancer care in this select patient group. The former defines a registered impact of age-related comorbidity, which has been shown to be particularly common in this patient cohort and includes the end-organ impact of hypertension, diabetes, atherosclerotic disease, chronic respiratory disease, and arthritis.[6,7] However, the number of comorbidities and their severity may not be entirely sufficient to adequately define frailty.[8]

This kind of objective assessment must in the elderly be considered against the frequent background of suboptimal surgical and adjuvant treatments in solid cancer management[9–11] and a reluctance by specialist clinicians to incorporate older patients either into clinical trials using novel chemotherapeutic and immunotherapeutic regimens or into existing screening programs,[12–14] where the barriers encountered to inclusion of the elderly include variations in physician perception regarding the safety of surgical therapies, protocol eligibility criteria, comorbidity exclusions,

[a] Department of Surgery and Transplantation, Chaim Sheba Medical Center, Tel-Aviv, Israel 52621
[b] University of Liverpool, St Helens Teaching Hospital, Marshalls Cross Road, St Helens WA9 3DA, UK
* Corresponding author.
E-mail address: apzbar1355@yahoo.com

Clin Geriatr Med 28 (2012) 51–71
doi:10.1016/j.cger.2011.09.002
0749-0690/12/$ – see front matter © 2012 Elsevier Inc. All rights reserved.

assumptions regarding the potential tolerability of treatments, and the perceived lack of social support networks necessary for optimal follow-up or for the ability to withstand treatment-related side effects requiring such support. These issues are intricate and may necessitate more specialized clinical trials in surgery that are age dependent, taking into account differences in tumor biology and treatment tolerance to modified or "tailored" régimes specifically designed for differently aged subsets.

There seems to be intrinsic biological differences in growth patterns, hormonal receptor expression, DNA ploidy, and tumor angiogenesis in many solid tumors, such as breast, prostate, and lung cancers, in the elderly when compared with younger-aged patient cohorts,[15] reflecting a more prolonged carcinogen exposure on a background of age-related immunosenescence potentially favoring cancer development and growth.[16–19] It is not clear how this biological difference might impact on treatment planning. Despite these inherent differences, in selected patients, there is ample evidence that cancer-specific outcome is equivalent regardless of age in a range of solid tumors when patients undergo resection with curative intent, including breast cancer,[20] colorectal cancer (CRC),[21] esophagogastric cancer,[22,23] and head and neck tumors,[24] but where there is relatively poor categorization of perioperative risk and an underutilization of surgically optimal resectional practice or adjuvant or neoadjuvant therapies.[25,26] This review discusses the general assessment instruments available for elderly cancer patients along with the issues involved in the more common site-specific cancers that pertain to this unique patient cohort.

COMPREHENSIVE GERIATRIC ASSESSMENT IN CANCER

A series of structured questionnaires have been recently established and validated for elderly patients with solid malignancies undergoing surgery incorporating the specific functional, mental, and social parameters that uniquely affect cancer-related outcome in this unique patient group.[27] In this regard, Audisio and colleagues in collaboration with the International Society of Geriatric Oncology and with geriatricians have developed the Preoperative Assessment of Cancer in the Elderly (PACE) questionnaire for rapid patient risk determination showing that 83% of patients have at least 1 relatively important comorbid condition and that two thirds of cases have acceptable functional and mental status preoperatively.[28,29] After adjustment for age, gender, and type of cancer, most of the PACE parameters have been shown to be significantly associated with other comorbidity indices (such as the Satariano Index of Comorbidity), where a multivariate analysis has identified that an instrumental activity of daily living index, fatigue, and the American Society of Anesthesia (ASA) grade are independent factors predicting for poor postoperative outcomes.[30–34] It is recognized, however, that the ASA grade for specific cancers such as CRC is not sufficiently sensitive in the prediction of operative risk between these 2 different groups where most elderly patients are classified as ASA grade II or III.[35,36] It is anticipated that a more intensive geriatric assessment will define a better estimate of remaining life expectancy, functional reserve, and treatment tolerance, as well as assisting in outlining individual barriers to perioperative management, adjuvant treatment planning, and hospital discharge.

These parameters are of major clinical importance where preoperative disturbances of the instrumental activity of daily living index, fatigue, and performance status lead to a 50% increase in the incidence of both postoperative complications[37] and hospital stay. Incorporating these questionnaires prospectively into multidimensional assessments will provide comparability of cancer-specific outcome data between elderly and younger patient cohorts in specific cancers and will assist in the identification of variability in preoperative staging and factors that limit the use of postoperative adjuvant therapies. Future studies will validate the use of other assessment systems, including PREOP, which are simpler and faster data acquisition tools than PACE and which incorporate the Groeningen Frailty Index,[38] the Vulnerable Elders Survey,[39] and the timed "up and go test."[40] The Groeningen Frailty Index is a 15-item questionnaire with simple 0/1 scores where a patient score of more than 3 indicates frailty and identifies patients with the potential for a decline in self-management capability. In this respect, the Groeningen Frailty Index score separates frail from nonfrail cases undergoing surgery for solid cancers in terms of physical, role, emotional, and social functioning in accordance with the criteria used in the assessment of health-related quality of life adopted by the European Organization of Research and Treatment in Cancer, which is part of their C-30 questionnaire used in a range of cancers including colorectal and head and neck cancers.[41,42]

Although these instruments require further validation and dissection, frailty as an index has been independently shown in a study from The Netherlands to be a major risk factor for institutionalization, mortality, and a decline in physical functioning after major cancer surgery in population-based patient cohorts.[43] Its discriminatory ability in the identification of patients with a heightened vulnerability to adverse health events indicative of multisystem reductions in functional reserve capacity is at present controversial.[44] The Vulnerable Elders Survey–13 is a 13-item questionnaire that addresses self-reported health issues and identifies vulnerable, older patients predicting as its own frailty index patients likely to undergo significant functional decline over the short term,[39] although it remains to be tested in the context of cancer surgery. The "up and go" test[40] measures physical performance status and represents a very simple criterion, such as the time taken to get out of a chair, to walk 3 m, and then return to the chair; as such, it remains to be validated as a prognostic variable in elderly patients undergoing cancer surgery.

BREAST CANCER

It has been well established that the survival outcome after breast-conserving surgery when used is independent of age,[45] although there seem to be significant clinician-related biases to information regarding breast conservation in older patients where the medical health alone is not a sufficient explanation for this group's high relative rate of mastectomy (**Table 1**).[46] In this respect, comorbid conditions are effectively not a contraindication toward breast-conserving surgery.[47] In frail patients, it has been clearly shown by the Group for Research on Endocrine Therapy in the Elderly trial that the progression rate of the primary where tamoxifen-only therapy is used is inferior to local excision combined with tamoxifen.[48] Other groups have also confirmed these findings comparing treatment with tamoxifen alone to mastectomy[49–51] or wide local excision,[52] where Fennessy and colleagues,[53] in a study of 455 patients aged 70 years and older, showed that surgery plus tamoxifen conferred a nonsignificant benefit in terms of overall survival but a significant improvement in local recurrence rates. In this respect, a Cochrane meta-analysis has reported that tamoxifen therapy alone is inferior to surgery (with or without tamoxifen) in terms of local tumor control and progression free survival in medically fit older women,[54] although there is no clear benefit for overall survival. The potential advantages of aromatase inhibitor therapy in similar trials are unknown in older frail patients with limited life expectancy where the outcome of surgery is unlikely be affect cancer-specific survival rates.

A further clear example of an age bias to adequate surgical treatment may be found in the variability of management of the axilla in older patients, where 2 large studies have analyzed databases in early stage invasive breast cancer. These include the

Table 1
Outcome studies of breast cancer in the elderly

Author	Year	Number	Study	LRR	OS
Robertson et al[49]	1988	68 Tamox alone 67 Mastectomy	R R	53 70	ND 24 mos
Grube et al[45]	2001	860 <70 yrs 190 >70 yrs	R	NS	91%, 3 yrs 93%, 3 yrs
Mustacchi et al[48]	2003 235 Tamox alone	239 Tamox + surgery	RCT	27 PD 106 PD	ND 3 yrs
Fentiman et al[51]	2003	82 Tamox alone 82 mastectomy	RTC	Reduced TTP	ND 10 years
Fennessy et al[53]	2004	230 Tamox alone 225 Surgery + Tamox	RCT	Reduced TTF	Divergence after 3 yrs
ALND					
Truong et al[25]	2002	8038	R	Similar ALND + or −	Reduced OS in older AD−
Martelli et al[62]	2005	219 Stage 1	RCT ALND+ ALND−	ND	ND at 60 mos
Rudenstam et al[63]	2007	234 Stage 1 Sx + ALND 230 Stage 1 Sx alone	RCT	ND	ND at 6.6 yrs

Abbreviations: ALND, axillary lymph node dissection; ND, no difference; PD, progressive disease; R, retrospective study; RCT, randomized controlled trial; Sx, surgery; TTF, time to failure; TTP, time to progression.

Breast Cancer Outcome database of 8038 women and the National Cancer database assessing 47,944 patients where the omission of appropriate axillary lymph node dissection (ALND) increased with advancing age.[55–57] In this regard, Bland and associates[56] showed that it was omitted in up to 60% of cases where it was deemed appropriate in patients over 80 years of age. This surgical omission has been based on the widely held view that total lymph node positivity in older patients is lower and that they have a less aggressive tumor diathesis,[58] although this is controversial; Gennari and colleagues[59] reported that elderly women were more likely to present with pathologically involved axillary lymph nodes compared with younger postmenopausal patients. The true value of ALND in clinically N0 elderly patients is nevertheless obscure; a recent study from Milan by Martelli and colleagues[60] showed no advantage, confirming the findings of the ACOSOG Z011 trial, where the omission of ALND did not impact on local recurrence, distant recurrence, or overall survival in older patient cohorts.

A further influencing factor away from more routine ALND is the presumption that older patients have a higher rate of postoperative lymphoedema,[61] although this too is controversial; Bland and co-workers[56] showed in a large patient cohort (84,877 women treated for stage I breast cancer) that in every clinical scenario involving breast-conserving surgery where ALND was omitted, there was a significantly lower rate of survival and that the addition of systemic therapy did not overcome the adverse effect of ALND omission. There does not seem to be any advantage for ALND in early T1N0 tumors in older patients for overall mortality, breast cancer-specific mortality, or the crude cumulative incidence of breast events (including local recurrence or metachronous cancer), where the incidence of axillary recurrence appears to be very low if a full ALND is not performed[62,63] and where sentinel lymph node biopsy in the elderly has been shown to be just as effective as in younger patient cohorts.[64]

The negative impact of undertreatment based on age is not only limited to surgical decisions, but also to restrictions on systemic and hormonal therapies,[65] despite the fact that there is little available evidence that elderly patients experience an increased risk of adverse chemotherapy-related events when such therapy is properly administered.[66] This issue is complex, however where; it is known that the risk of hospitalization for chemotherapy-related events, although unaffected by age, is associated with higher rates of dehydration, anaemia, and neutropenia in older patients, which can be managed in an ambulatory setting.[67]

Recommendations

- Hormonal treatment alone in elderly patients is inferior to surgery plus hormonal treatment.
- Operative approaches in frail elderly patients should be similar, given the low attendant morbidity and mortality.
- ALND is underutilized in elderly patients when indicated.
- Sentinel lymph node biopsy should be routinely used in older patients.

HEAD AND NECK CANCERS

Head and neck cancer represents the 6th commonest malignancy and the 8th leading cause of cancer mortality worldwide, with one quarter of cases occurring in patients over the age of 70 years[68] and where age-adjusted outcomes have been shown to be equivalent to younger cohorts in cancers of the thyroid and larynx as well as in a mixed range of head and neck tumors.[69–72] In this broad context, head and neck cancers include malignancies arising in the paranasal sinuses, nasal and oral cavity, pharynx, and larynx; the oral cavity, larynx, and oropharynx are the commonest sites of malignancy in elderly cases.[73] There is an increased proportion of females in older cohorts than occurs in younger patients.[74] In these circumstances, half the mortality is related to pulmonary complications[75]; associated medical conditions have a high prevalence in this group, including alcohol abuse and heavy smoking.[76] This has led to a modification of the Kaplan–Feinstein comorbidity index to a specialized comorbidity evaluation widely utilized in elderly head and neck cases.[77,78] Latterly, the McPeek postoperative outcome score has been utilized to evaluate the success of major extirpative surgical intervention in elderly head and neck cancer where neither age nor ASA score independently predicted comorbidity, duration of surgery, or postoperative performance.[79]

It is accepted that few randomized, controlled trials have incorporated patients over 65 years of age in newer treatment modalities and radiotherapeutic delivery systems[80–82]; it is known that squamous cell cancer of the head and neck tends to present in a more locally advanced stage but with fewer neck node metastases when compared with younger patients[83] and up to one third of older patients have a simultaneous second primary malignancy.[73] Differences in perception of rehabilitation and reconstruction seem to be age dependent, where oral prosthetics are reliant on improved dental implantation, dependent on preoperative bone stock.[84–86] There are no currently available trial data where specific rehabilitation regimes and reconstructive techniques have been made specifically available to elderly patients and where age itself is an isolated and specific factor in the perioperative management protocol.[87]

Age as such does not affect the locoregional recurrence rates or disease-free survival in head and neck cancers,[88] with the higher comorbidity in older cases not actually influencing the reported incidence of postoperative complications.[89,90] In older patients, concurrent illnesses and operation duration influence the overall complication rate of flap reconstructions and the length of hospital stay, but there is no overall impact of age when these surgeries are used,[91–95] although this is affected by individually tailored anesthesia, where there are differences in the pharmacokinetics and pharmacodynamics of anesthetic agents and unique airway issues.[96] The likelihood of complications is more dependent on male gender, the use of bilateral radical neck dissection, those patients with more than 2 recorded comorbidities, clinical stage IV disease, and the utilization of reconstructive surgery than it is per se on chronologic age.[76]

As in surgery, age may create individual biases in radiation protocols as well as in the selective use of chemotherapy. In this respect, the range of radiotherapeutic techniques used makes unequivocal statements concerning the elderly difficult, even in tumors such as early glottis cancers, those of the base of the tongue, and tonsillar lesions, where radiation is utilized as the principal treatment modality for cure. Here, hyperfractionation has shown advantage over accelerated fractionation in improving local tumor control and providing a marginal survival benefit at the expense of a small increase in side effects, although the large European Organization of Research and Treatment in Cancer trials (22,851 and 22,791) examining its benefits did not stratify patients for age,[97,98] where meta-analysis has shown a lower compliance and tolerance in older cases.[99] Although age itself does not represent a true radiotherapeutic limitation, there are several confounding variables in its assessment and clinical impact.[100,101] These include differences in reporting of radiation with curative or palliative intent in many studies of the upper aerodigestive tract,[24,80] where patients are strictly not comparable and where the elderly show a rapid initial survival drop postoperatively, regardless of disease stage. Here studies incorporate a mixture of cancer types, different radiation protocols and doses with different intents and use of these different regimes in different disease stages[102] with variable effects on local control and disease-free survival of treatment interruption or on the place for accelerated boost schedules in the extreme old patient subgroup.[103] Further, there are limited data concerning severe toxicity in the elderly where 1 study reporting 1589 patients of whom 20% were over 65 years of age showed no effect of age on acute mucosal toxicity, although there were age-related differences in severe grade functional disability in the short term.[82]

The place of chemotherapy is expanding, although in the literature curative and palliative goals of therapy should be differentiated. In those cases where disease is unresectable, where organ preservation is a priority, where R1 resections are performed, or where there is extracapsular spread, age should not affect the decision for chemotherapy. Comparison of reports is difficult where neoadjuvant/induction strategies, adjuvant protocols, and concomitant regimes are frequently not separated. Here, nonrandomized data suggest a greater chemotherapeutic benefit under the age of 60 years with less acute and delayed toxicity and dental problems.[82] The role in these patients of newer agents (including docetaxel as an induction agent with carboplatin-based regimes or paclitaxel—the current E1393/5 trials) as it specifically

Table 2
Outcome studies of esophageal cancer in the elderly

Author	Year	Number	Study	% Complications	LOS
Jougon et al[123]	1997	89 > 70 yrs 451 < 70 yrs	R	NS	ND
Alexiou et al[124]	1998	186 > 70 yrs 337 < 70 yrs	R	36 25[a]	ND
Sabel et al[125]	2002	147 > 70 yrs 266 < 70 yrs	R	ND	ND
Bonavina et al[126]	2003	403 > 70 yrs 497 < 70 yrs	R	ND	ND
Ruol et al[127]	2007	159 > 70 yrs 580 < 70 yrs	R	ND	ND
Shimada et al[129]	2007	55 > 70 yrs 65 < 70 yrs	R	ND	ND
Morita et al[130]	2008	184 > 70 yrs 494 < 70 yrs	R	ND	NS
Takeno et al[131]	2008	25 > 80 yrs 95 < 80 yrs	R	ND	ND
Elsayed et al[133]	2010	218 > 70 yrs 108 < 70 yrs	R	12% mortality 5% mortality[a]	ND
Yang et al[134]	2010	136 > 70 yrs 136 < 70 yrs	R	5.9% mortality 0.7% mortality[a]	ND
Zehetner et al[135]	2010	47 > 80 yrs 513 < 80 yrs	R	ND	ND
Cijs et al[122]	2010	250 > 70 yrs 811 < 70 yrs	R	17 20	27% at 5 yrs 34% at 5 yrs[a]

Abbreviations: ND, no difference; NS, not stated; R, retrospective study.
[a] Statistical difference.

pertains to older patients is currently poorly documented where initial results suggest that the elderly have similar objective response rates and times to disease progression in locally advanced and inoperable cases albeit at the expense of greater toxicity, most notably, nephrotoxicity, diarrhea, and thrombocytopenia, and a greater requirement for supplementary colony-stimulating factor therapy.[104]

Recommendations

- Extensive resections are feasible in the elderly, although there is greater postoperative respiratory morbidity and mortality.
- Radiotherapy and adjuvant chemotherapy are equally well tolerated in the elderly when compared with younger patient cohorts.
- Complex reconstruction may be offered to elderly patients.

ESOPHAGOGASTRIC CANCER

The overall prevalence rates of gastric cancer are decreasing, although there are a disparate number of elderly cases where one third of gastric cancers occur in patients 70 years or older (**Table 2**).[105] The outcomes in older patients are similar to those achieved in younger cohorts,[106] although it is accepted that D2 resections with less extensive lymphadenectomy tends to be performed in older patients without any specific effect on survival.[107] These patients have, however, a higher medium- and long-term non-cancer mortality[108] without any effect on perceived quality of life.[109] This approach also applies to total gastrectomy if indicated by site.[110,111] Currently, Comprehensive Geriatric Assessment (CGA) analysis data are unavailable in the elderly for upper gastrointestinal tumors, where it is known that there is a higher prevalence of hypertension, electrocardiographic anomalies, altered nutritional status, and coincident pulmonary disease.[112,113] Although it is clear that older patients have similar outcomes to younger cohorts in nonrandomized series undergoing gastrectomy with curative intent, there is bias in survival analyses where older age, lymph node involvement, T3 and T4 disease, and higher tumor grade are linked with outcomes[114] and where there is no clear survival benefit with adjuvant chemotherapy. In this setting, the initial survival advantage seems to be conferred in older patients by a laparoscopic approach,[115,116] although there are few prospective, randomized data that assesses the method of surgery in different age groups. For the older cohort, where the incidence of proximal gastric carcinoma has shown a rise in recent years, there is an initial toll of total gastrectomy with equivalent benefits in survivors,[117,118] and a recent meta-analysis has shown conflicting data concerning D1 versus D2 gastrectomy in terms of hospital stay, complications, anastomotic leakage, and the need for reoperation.[119] Data currently pertaining to the best operative, neoadjuvant, and postoperative adjuvant approaches for the elderly with gastric carcinoma are lacking, with little available evidence concerning the benefit of comprehensive geriatric assessment in selected cases.[120,121]

There are a number of studies assessing esophageal resection for cancer in the elderly; most show a substantial increase in cardiovascular and respiratory concomitant disease and some showing a higher prevalence of underlying Barrett's mucosa with malignant transformation.[122] There seems to be a similar outcome in selected cases with a similar incidence of surgical complications but a higher prevalence of nonsurgical postoperative complications and in some series a higher operative and in-hospital mortality along with a lower 1-year survival reflecting the impact of these factors on early death.[123–134] In many studies, tumors are more advanced in the elderly with less use of neoadjuvant therapy and reduced selective use of transhiatal resection.[135] The selective utilization of neoadjuvant therapies in older patients does not seem to be associated with an increased morbidity or postoperative mortality.[128,136]

Recommendations

- Esophagectomy is as well tolerated in the elderly as in younger cohorts.
- Resection in older patients is often associated with a higher preoperative comorbidity and consequently a higher respiratory- and cardiovascular-related perioperative mortality in some series.
- Lower initial survival is associated with equivalent long-term survival rates even when total gastrectomy (where indicated) is included as part of postoperative management.

COLORECTAL CANCER

Original collated data from the Association of Coloproctology of Great Britain and Ireland suggested that there was an age-adjusted increase in mortality in CRC with patients between 65 and 74 years having a 1.8 times greater likelihood of death, those between 75 and 84 years a 3.5-fold increase, and those older than 85 years, a 5-fold increase in death rate after elective colorectal resection (**Table 3**).[137] These data were,

Table 3
Outcome studies of colorectal cancer in the elderly

Author	Year	Number	Study	% Complications	OS
Colon cancer					
Chiappa et al[169]	2005	479 < 70 yrs	R	1.4% Mortality	54% at 5 yrs
		213 > 70 yrs		0.8% Mortality	67%[a]
Richter et al[163]	2005	1000 < 70 yrs	R	NR	ND at 5 yrs
		332 > 70 yrs			
Pavlidis et al[141]	2006	105	R	Morbidity 25%	
Isobe et al[165]	2007	130 < 80 yrs	R	Increased	ND
		67 > 80 yrs		delirium	
Chautard et al[151]	2008	103 < 70 yrs	L	NS morbidity	NR
		75 > 70 yrs			
Basili et al[166]	2008	115 < 70 yrs	R	0% Mortality	NR
		134 > 70 yrs		3.4%[a]	
Fiscon et al[153]	2010	134 < 75 yrs	L	NS	NR
		82 > 75 yrs			
Pinto et al[152]	2011	> 80 yrs	L		
		116 Open		3.4% Mortality	
		83 Laparoscopic		2.4%	
Rectal cancer					
Hotta et al[173]	2007	33 > 75 yrs	R	ND	
		125 < 75 yrs			
Akiyoshi et al[181]	2009	44 > 75 yrs	L/R	NS	
		228 < 75 yrs			
Kurian et al[185]	2011	Patients > 80 yrs	R		
		99 Emergent		28% Mortality	
		63 Elective		4.7%[a]	
Frasson et al[187]	2008	334 < 70 yrs	R	23.9% Morbidity	
		201		37.5%[a]	

Abbreviations: L, laparoscopy versus open; ND, no difference; NR, not reported; R, retrospective study.
[a] Significant difference detected.

however, not adjusted for ASA grade, cancer site, or stage, although the issues are complex; the Colorectal Cancer Collaborative Group has previously shown that older patients with CRC have a higher baseline comorbidity, more advanced disease stage, and undergo more frequent emergency surgery.[138] In this respect, elderly patients present as colorectal emergencies (obstruction and perforation) in up to 40% of cases, with a higher incidence of palliative surgery and a lower utilization of adjuvant and neoadjuvant therapies.[139,140]

The issues (and opportunities) available to all patients with CRC should be part of oncologic practice in the elderly, including access to laparoscopic and robotic technology, emergency stenting (where appropriate), and utilization of adjuvant and neoadjuvant therapies. Older patients presenting with obstructive CRC have a death rate 3 times higher than that of younger cohorts presenting as colonic emergencies where typically the older case undergoes a diverting stoma[141] and where at least half the patients will never undergo stoma reversal. There are no current available data where age is an independent factor concerning outcome of stented versus unstented patients where studies have been nonrandomized or where comparisons have been made with palliative surgery only and where the indications for use (bridge approach versus definitive approach) have not been adequately compared.[142,143]

In the bridging situation, successful primary anastomosis rates seem to be higher among the stented group with an acceptably low leakage rate (3% with a stent versus 11% with no stent), along with a shorter hospital stay and reduced surgical intensive care unit utilization,[143] although there is little available information concerning the effect of a bridge on overall cancer-specific outcomes.[144] The exact place of stenting remains controversial where the complication rate (late perforation) has been unexpectedly high in the Dutch Stent-in-1 trial necessitating early trial closure.[145,146] Cost analyses comparing stents with surgery have shown that stenting results in 23% fewer operative procedures per patient (1.01 vs 1.32 operations per patient) with an 83% reduction in stoma formation (7% vs 43% and a lower procedure-related mortality (5% vs 11%) and a lower mean cost per patient where stenting options were used first.[147] The most recent data from China comparing mortality, stoma avoidance, and short-term survival specifically in the elderly where stents were compared with acute surgery matched for tumor distribution and comorbidity showed a successful stent deployment rate of 91% with a higher rate of primary anastomosis (79% vs 47%; $P = .002$) and a comparable mortality and morbidity between groups.[148] There is much work yet to be done with age an independent factor in the decision making for acute stents, particularly because the site of the obstruction does not seem to play a factor[149] and because longer term palliation is best achieved in colonic cases rather than in tumors creating extracolonic obstruction.[150]

Recent, comparative data clearly show advantage for older patients in the laparoscopic approach, akin to younger cases with significantly less blood loss when compared with open surgery and an overall faster recovery,[151,152] and without any specific age-related effect on perioperative mortality[153] or short- or medium-term outcomes.[154] The utilization of laparoscopic surgery in potentially more advanced cancers presenting in older patients requires larger studies,[155] where there might be a higher incidence of preclusive prior abdominal surgery[156] and differential adverse effects of laparoscopic conversion.[157] Collective series have repeatedly shown that the short-term morbidity and survival are equivalent in elderly patients undergoing elective colorectal resection when compared with younger cohorts.[141,158–166] There is also considerable evidence to suggest that, when chemotherapy is indicated, elderly patients receive suboptimal treatment[167]; its more routine and standardized use is associated an acceptable quality of life, completion of therapy, and cost.[168–170]

In rectal cancer, the principal issues include the more routine use of neoadjuvant therapy and laparoscopic surgery. Nonrandomized data suggest that neoadjuvant treatment is well tolerated regardless of age[171,172] where age is an independent risk factor for overall survival but not for disease-free survival[173] and where response seems to be lower if the tumor is located in the mid rectum, where radiation doses are less than 40 cGy and where it is not combined with chemotherapy.[174] Overall combined toxicity seems to be similar in older patients, although there is some correlation with comorbidity and a slightly higher incidence of hematologic toxicity.[175–177] Like younger patients, in the specialist group where there is total chemoradiotherapeutic response in early (c0) tumors with a watchful waiting policy, systemic early failure (as opposed to salvageable local recurrence) seems to be the main limiting factor.[178] Neoadjuvant treatment may also provide a reasonable window of opportunity to offer appropriate pre-habilitation to older cancer patients improving their general condition and nutrition as well as impacting on preoperative depression, anemia, and electrolyte balance.

With regard to the extended role of laparoscopic and robotic surgery in the elderly, there is a paucity of data. Perioperative morbidity is affected by the inherent operative learning curve,[179] as well as by the higher comorbidity observed in older patients.[180] In one of the few available studies assessing the impact of age on elective laparoscopic rectal surgery, Akiyoshi and colleagues[181] compared 44 patients over the age of 75 years with 228 younger patients undergoing elective laparoscopic rectal resection as well as with 43 elderly patients having open rectal resections, and showed no differences between the laparoscopic groups in terms of operating times, estimated blood loss, or postoperative complication rates, but a marked reduction in blood loss compared with the open group, despite a substantial increase in operating time when the laparoscopic approach was adopted. Although in this study the incidence of postoperative complications was lower in the elderly laparoscopic group compared with the open elderly group, these differences did not attain significance. The implication is that laparoscopic procedures should not be denied to appropriate patients because of their chronologic age. Further, it is anticipated that tumor size, operator experience, and tumor location as well as intrinsic "pelvic" factors such as gender and body habitus and mass index are more important than age-,related nonsurgical factors in determining the success rate of laparoscopic rectal resection.[182] Equally, the likelihood of conversion during laparoscopic rectal resection is greater in cancer compared with diverticular disease, where estimated blood loss during laparoscopic excision is less pronounced in cases of Crohn's resections, suggestive of the inherent factors implicated in operative difficulty (however that is performed), which lie outside age-dependent criteria.[183] In nonrandomized, open-label data from an elderly cohort undergoing elective laparoscopic colorectal resection, Robinson and colleagues[154] showed that patients undergoing the minimally invasive approach had earlier return to bowel function and a reduced length of hospital stay with fewer postoperative cardiac complications and equivalent survival when compared with open surgery. Both groups showed similar circumferential resection margins and extent of lymphadenectomy.[184]

Further factors involved in patient outcome, which are more age dependent, show a greater incidence of postoperative renal failure and in-hospital deaths where surgery is emergent in elderly patients and where social considerations such as admission to hospital from a nursing facility correlated with higher rates of in-hospital mortality.[185] In these patients, it is accepted that the length of the procedure in these circumstances, the presence of significant postoperative complications, and the need for perioperative blood transfusion predict 6-month postoperative mortality. Although there are limited data, those considered traditionally high risk may receive more benefit from this approach.[186,187]

Recommendations

- Survival statistics in older cohorts of CRC resection with curative intent are equivalent to younger patients.
- The higher incidence of emergency CRC resections accounts for a substantial increase in CRC perioperative mortality.
- Postoperative adjuvant therapy is well tolerated in elderly patient cohorts.
- Laparoscopic surgery has selective advantage in both rectal and colonic resection in the elderly.
- Neoadjuvant therapy for rectal cancer has equivalent indications and tolerance in elderly patients and may permit pre-habilitation.
- The use of stents in the emergency setting may be advisable.

SUMMARY

Elderly patients constitute the largest group in oncologic medical practice, despite the fact that in solid cancers treated operatively, many patients are denied standard therapies and where such decision making is based solely on age. The "natural" assumptions that we have are often misleading; namely, that the elderly cannot tolerate complex or difficult procedures, chemotherapy, or radiation schedules; that their overall predictable medical health determines survival (and not the malignancy); or that older patients typically have less aggressive tumors. Clearly, patient selection and a comprehensive geriatric assessment is key where well-selected cases have the same cancer-specific survival as younger cohorts in a range of tumors as outlined including upper and lower gastrointestinal malignancy, head and neck cancer, and breast cancer.[188,189]

The assessment of patient fitness for surgery and adjuvant therapies is therefore critical to outcomes,[190] where studies have clearly shown that fit older patients experience the same benefits and toxicities of chemotherapy as do younger patients and that when normalized for preexisting medical conditions, that older patients tolerate major operative procedures designed with curative oncological intent. At present, our problem is the lack of true evidence-based medicine specifically designed with age in mind, which effectively limits surgical decision making in disease-based strategies. This can only be achieved by the utilization of more standardized, comprehensive geriatric assessments to identify vulnerable older patients, aggressive pre-habilitation with amelioration of vulnerability causation, improvement of patient-centered longitudinal outcomes, and an improved surgical and medical understanding of relatively subtle decreases in organ functioning, social support mechanisms and impairments of health-related quality of life as a feature specifically of advanced age.[36,191–193]

REFERENCES

1. Jernal A, Murray T, Samuels A, et al. Cancer statistics 2003. CA Cancer J Clin 2003;53:5–26.
2. Davis DL, Dinse GE, Hoel DG. Decreasing cardiovascular disease and increasing cancer among whites in the United States from 1973 through 1987: good news and bad news. JAMA 1984;271:431–7.
3. Leading causes of death in the United States, 1973 vs 1999. J Natl Cancer Inst 2002;94:1742.
4. Projections of the total resident population by 5-year age groups and sex with special age categories. Middle Series 2025–2045. Washington (DC): Population Projection Program Population Division US Census Bureau; 2000. Publication no. NP-T3-F.
5. Gómez Portilla A, Martínez de Lecea C, Cendoya I, et al. Prevalence and treatment of oncologic disease in the elderly: an impending challenge. Rev Esp Enferm Dis 2008;11:706–15.
6. Yancik R, Havlik RJ, Wesley MN, et al. Cancer and comorbidity in older patients: a descriptive profile. Ann Epidemiol 1996;6:399–412.
7. Ogle KS, Swanson GM, Woods N, et al. Cancer and comorbidity: redefining chronic diseases. Cancer 2000;88:653–63.
8. Read WL, Tierney RL, Page NC, et al. Differential prognostic impact of comorbidity. J Clin Oncol 2004;22:3099–103.
9. Sekue I, Fukuda X, Kumitoh H, et al. Cancer chemotherapy in the elderly. Jpn J Clin Oncol 1998;28:463–73.

10. Wasil T, Lichtman SM, Gupta V, et al. Radiation therapy in cancer patients 80 years of age or older. Am J Clin Oncol 2000;23:526–30.
11. Audisio RA, Bozzetti F, Gennari R, et al. The surgical management of elderly cancer patients: recommendations of the SIOG surgical task force. Eur J Cancer 2004;40: 926–38.
12. Trimble EL, Carter CL, Cain D, et al. Representation of older patients in cancer treatment trials. Cancer 1994;74:2208–14.
13. Townsley CA, Selby R, Siu LL. Systematic review of barriers to the recruitment of older patients with cancer onto clinical trials. J Clin Oncol 2005;23:3112–24.
14. Aapro MS, Köhne CH, Cohen HJ, et al. Never too old? Age should not be a barrier to enrollment in cancer clinical trials. Oncologist 2005;10:198–204.
15. Piantanelli L. Cancer and aging: from the kinetics of biological parameters and the kinetics of cancer incidence and mortality. Ann N Y Acad Sci 1988;521:99–101.
16. Anisimov VN. Biology of aging and cancer. Cancer Control 2007;14:23–31.
17. Malaguarnera I, Ferlito L, DiMauro S, et al. Immunosenescence and cancer: a review. Arch Gerontol Geriatr 2001;32:77–93.
18. Whiteside TL. Cell-mediated dysregulation in malignancy and its therapeutic immunopotentiation. In: Zbar AP, Bland KI, Syrigos KN, et al, editors. Immunology for surgeons. London: Springer-Verlag; 2002. p. 263–80.
19. Fulop T, Larbi A, Kotb R, et al. Aging, immunity, and cancer. Discov Med 2011;11: 537–50.
20. Wildiers H, Kunkler I, Biganzoli L, et al; International Society of Geriatric Oncology. Management of breast cancer in elderly individuals: recommendations of the International Society of Geriatric Oncology. Lancet Oncol 2007;8:1101–15.
21. Papamichael D, Audisio R, Horiot JC, et al; SIOG. Treatment of the elderly colorectal cancer patient: SIOG expert recommendations. Ann Oncol 2009;20:5–16.
22. Gretschel S, Estevez-Schwarz L, Hunerbein M, et al. Gastric cancer surgery in elderly patients. World J Surg 2006;30:1468–74.
23. Chang AC, Lee JS. Resection for esophageal cancer in the elderly. Thorac Surg Clin 2009;19:333–43.
24. Bernardi D, Barzan L, Franchin G, et al. Treatment of head and neck cancer in elderly patients: state of the art and guidelines. Crit Rev Oncol Hematol 2005;53:71–80.
25. Truong PT, Bernstein V, Wai E, et al. Age-related variations in the use of axillary dissection: a survival analysis of 8038 women with T1-ST2 breast cancer. Int J Radiat Oncol Biol Phys 2002;54:794–803.
26. Neugut AI, Fleischauer AT, Sundararajan V, et al. Use of adjuvant chemotherapy and radiation therapy for rectal cancer among the elderly: a population-based study. J Clin Oncol 2002;20:2643–50.
27. Maas HA, Janssen-Heijnen ML, Olde Rikkert MG, et al. Comprehensive geriatric assessment and its clinical impact in oncology. Eur J Cancer 2007;43:2161–9.
28. Pope D, Ramesh H, Gennari R, et al. Pre-operative assessment of cancer in the elderly (PACE): a comprehensive assessment of underlying characteristics of elderly cancer patients prior to elective surgery. Surg Oncol 2006;15:189–97.
29. PACE participants. Shall we operate? Preoperative assessment in elderly cancer patients (PACE can help. A SIOG surgical task force prospective study. Crit Rev Oncol Hematol 2008;65:156–63.
30. New classification of physical status. American society of anaesthesiologists. Anesthesiology 1963;24:111.
31. Lawton MP, Brody EM. Assessment of older people: self-maintaining and instrumental activities of daily living. Gerontologist 1969;9:179–86.

32. Satariano WA, Ragland DR. The effect of comorbidity on 3-year survival of women with primary breast cancer. Ann Intern Med 1994;120:104–10.
33. Mendoza TR, Wang XS, Cleeland CS, et al. The rapid assessment of fatigue severity in cancer patients: use of the brief fatigue inventory. Cancer 1999;85:1186–96.
34. Audisio RA, van Leeuwen B. When reporting on older patients with cancer, frailty information is needed. Ann Surg Oncol 2011;18:4–5.
35. Kristjansson SR, Nesbakken A, Jordhoy MS, et al. Comprehensive geriatric assessment can predict complications in elderly patients after elective surgery for colorectal cancer: a prospective observational cohort study. Crit Rev Oncol Hematol 2010;76:208–17.
36. Turrentine FE, Wang H, Simpson VB, et al. Surgical risk factors, morbidity and mortality in elderly patients. J Am Coll Surg 2006;203:865–77.
37. Kristjansson SR, Farinella E, Gaskell S, et al. Surgical risk and post-operative complications in older unfit cancer patients. Cancer Treat Rev 2009;35:499–502.
38. Slaets J. Vulnerability in the elderly: frailty. Med Clin North Am 2006;90:593–601.
39. Saliba D, Elliott M, Rubenstein LZ, et al. The vulnerable elders survey: a tool for identifying vulnerable older people in the community. J Am Geriatr Soc 2001;49:1691–9.
40. Podsiadlo D, Richardson S. The timed "up and go": a test of basic functional mobility for frail elderly persons. J Am Geriatr Soc 1991;39:142–8.
41. Aaronson NK, Ahmedzai S, Bergman B, et al. The European Organization for Research and Treatment of Cancer QLQ-C30: a national quality-of-life instrument for use in international clinical trials in oncology. J Nat Cancer Inst 1993;85:365–76.
42. Bjordal K, de Graeff A, Fayers PM, et al. A 12 country field study of the EORTC QLQ-C30 (version 3.0) and the head and neck cancer specific module (E ORTC QLQ-H&N35) in head and neck patients. EORTC Quality of Life Group. Eur J Cancer 2000;36:1796–807.
43. Schuurmans H, Steverink N, Lindenberg S, et al. Old or frail: what tells us more? J Gerontol A Biol Sci Med Sci 2004;59:M962–5.
44. Martin FC, Brighton P. Frailty: different tools for different purposes? Age Ageing 2008;37:129–31.
45. Grube BJ, Hansen NM, Ye W, et al. Surgical management of breast cancer in the elderly. Am J Surg 2001;182:359–64.
46. Liang W, Burnett CB, Rowland JH, et al. Communication between physicians and older women with localized breast cancer: implications for treatment and patient satisfaction. J Clin Oncol 2002;20:1008–16.
47. Morrow M, Bucci C, Rademaker A. Medical contraindications are not a major factor in the underutilization of breast conserving therapy. J Am Coll Surg 1998;186:269–74.
48. Mustacchi G, Ceccherini R, Milani S, et al. Italian Cooperative Group GRETA. Tamoxifen alone versus adjuvant Tamoxifen for operable breast cancer of the elderly: long term results of the phase III randomized controlled multicenter GRETA trial. Ann Oncol 2003;14:414–20.
49. Robertson JFR, Todd JH, Ellis IO, et al. Comparison of mastectomy with tamoxifen for treating elderly patients with operable breast cancer. Br Med J 1988;297:511–4.
50. Gazet JC, Ford HT, Coombes RC, et al. Prospective randomized trial of tamoxifen vs surgery in elderly patients with breast cancer. Eur J Surg Oncol 1994;20:207–14.
51. Fentiman IS, Christiaens MR, Paridaens R, et al. EORTC. Treatment of operable breast cancer in the elderly: a randomised clinical trial EORTC 10851 comparing tamoxifen alone with modified radical mastectomy. Eur J Cancer 2003;39:309–16.

52. Kenny FS, Robertson JFR, Ellis IO, et al. Long-term follow-up of elderly patients randomized to primary tamoxifen or wedge mastectomy as initial therapy for operable breast cancer. Breast 1998;7:35–9.
53. Fennessy M, Bates T, MacRae K, et al. Late follow-up of a randomized trial of surgery plus tamoxifen versus tamoxifen alone in women aged over 70 years with operable breast cancer. Br J Surg 2004;91:699–704.
54. Hind D, Wyld L, Reed MW. Surgery, with or without tamoxifen, versus tamoxifen alone for older women with operable breast cancer. Cochrane review. Br J Cancer 2007;96:1025–9.
55. Edge SB, Gold K, Berg CD, et al. Outcomes and Preferences for Treatment in Older Women Nationwide Study Research Team. Outcomes and preferences for treatment in older women nationwide study research team: patient and provider characteristics that affect the use of axillary dissection in older women with stage I-II breast carcinoma. Cancer 2002;94:2534–41.
56. Bland KI, Scottg-Conner CE, Menck H, et al. Axillary dissection in breast-conserving surgery for stage I and II breast cancer: a National Cancer Database Study of patterns of omission and implications for survival. J Am Coll Surg 1999;188:586–95.
57. Lupe K, Truong PT, Alexander C, et al. Ten-year locoregional recurrence risks in women with nodal micrometastatic breast cancer staged with axillary dissection. Int J Radiat Oncol Biol Phys 2011. [Epub ahead of print].
58. Fisher CJ, Egan MK, Smith P, et al. Histopathology of breast cancer in relation to age. Br J Cancer 1997;75:593–6.
59. Gennari R, Curigliano G, Rotmensz N. Breast carcinoma in elderly women: features of disease presentation, choice of local and systemic treatments compared with younger postmenopausal patients. Cancer 2004;101:1302–10.
60. Martelli G, Miceli R, Daidone MG, et al. Axillary dissection versus no axillary dissection in elderly patients with breast cancer and no palpable axillary nodes: results after 15 years of follow-up. Ann Surg Oncol 2011;18:125–38.
61. Mandelblatt JS, Edge SB, Meropol NJ, et al. Sequelae of axillary lymph node dissection in older women with stage 1 and 2 breast carcinoma. Cancer 2002;95: 2445–54.
62. Martelli G, Boracchi P, De Palo M, et al. A randomized trial comparing axillary dissection to no axillary dissection in older patients with T1N0 breast cancer: results after 5 years of follow-up. Ann Surg 2005;242:1–6.
63. International Breast Cancer Study Group; Rudenstam CM, Zahrieh D, Forbes JF, et al. Randomized trial comparing axillary clearance versus no axillary clearance in older patients with breast cancer: first results of the International Breast Cancer Study Group Trial 10-93. J Clin Oncol 2006;24:337–44.
64. Gennari R, Rotmensz N, Perego E, et al. Sentinel node biopsy in elderly breast cancer patients. Surg Oncol 2004;13:193–6.
65. Gajdos C, Tartter PI, Bleiweiss IJ, et al. The consequence of undertreating breast cancer in the elderly. J Am Coll Surg 2001;192:698–707.
66. Blackman SB, Lash TL, Fink AK, et al. Advanced age and adjuvant tamoxifen prescription in early-stage breast carcinoma patients. Cancer 2002;95:2465–72.
67. Du XL, Osborne C, Goodwin JS. Population-based assessment of hospitalizations for toxicity from chemotherapy in older women with breast cancer. J Clin Oncol 2002;20:4636–42.
68. Muir CS, Fraumeni JF Jr, Doll R. The interpretation of time trends. Cancer Surv 1994;1920:5–21.

69. Kowalski LP, Alcantara PS, Magrin J, et al. A case-control study on complications and survival in elderly patients undergoing major head and neck surgery. Am J Surg 1994;168:485–90.

70. Bliss R, Patel N, Guniea A, et al. Age is no contraindication to thyroid surgery. Age Ageing 1999;28:363–6.

71. Magnano M, De Stefani A, Usai A. Carcinoma of the larynx in the elderly: analysis of potentially significant prognostic variables. Aging 1999;11:316–22.

72. Boruk M, Chernobilsky BM, Rosenfeld RM, et al. Age as a prognostic factor for complications of major head and neck surgery. Arch Otolaryngol Head Neck Surg 2005;13:605–9.

73. Koch WM, Patel H, Brennan J, et al. Squamous cell carcinoma of the head and neck in the elderly. Arch Otolaryngol Head Neck Surg 1995;121:262–5.

74. Sarini J, Fournier C, Lefebvre JL, et al. Head and neck squamous cell carcinoma in elderly patients: a long-term retrospective review of 273 cases. Arch Otolaryngol Head Neck Surg 2001;127:1089–92.

75. Morgan RF, Hirata RM, Jaques DA, et al. Head and neck surgery in the aged. Am J Surg 1982;144:449–51.

76. Sanabria A, Carvalho AL, Vartanian JG, et al. Comorbidity is a prognostic factor in elderly patients with head and neck cancer. Ann Surg Oncol 2007;14:1449–57.

77. Piccirillo JF. Importance of comorbidity in head and neck cancer. Laryngoscope 2000;110:593–602.

78. Piccirillo JF, Tierney RM, Costas I, et al. Prognostic importance of comorbidity in a hospital-based cancer registry. J Am Med Assoc 2004;29:2441–7.

79. Sesterhenn AM, Schotte TL, Bauhofer A, et al. Head and neck cancer surgery in the elderly: outcome evaluation with the McPeek score. Ann Otol Rhinol Laryngol 2011;120:110–5.

80. Lusinchi A, Bourhis J, Wibault P, et al. Radiation therapy for head and neck cancers in the elderly. Int J Radiat Biol Phys 1990;18:819–23.

81. Metges JP, Eschwege F, de Crevoisier R, et al. Radiotherapy in head and neck cancer in the elderly: a challenge. Crit Rev Oncol Hematol 2000;34:195–203.

82. Syrigos KN, Karachalios D, Karapanagiotou EM, et al. Head and neck cancer in the elderly: an overview on the treatment modalities. Cancer Treat Rev 2009;35: 237–45.

83. Jones AS, Husband D, Rowley H. Radical radiotherapy for squamous cell carcinoma of the larynx, oropharynx and hypopharynx: patterns of recurrence, treatment and survival. Clin Otolaryngol Allied Sci 1998;23:496–511.

84. Logemann JA, Pauloski BR, Rademaker AW, et al. Speech and swallowing rehabilitation for head and neck cancer patients. Oncology (Williston Park) 1997;11:651–6, 659.

85. Sanders AD, Blom ED, Singer MI, et al. Reconstructive and rehabilitative aspects of head and neck cancer in the elderly. Otolaryngol Clin North Am 1990;23:1159–68.

86. Al Mardini M. Prosthetic rehabilitation of the head and neck: the state of the art. Curr Opin Otolaryngol Head Neck Surg 2009;17:253–7.

87. Smith RB, Sniezek JC, Weed DT, et al. Utilization of free tissue transfer in head and neck surgery. Otolaryngol Head Neck Surg 2007;137:182–91.

88. Jones AS, Goodyear PW, Ghosh S, et al. Extensive neck node metastases (N3) in head and neck squamous carcinoma: is radical treatment warranted? Otolaryngol Head Neck Surg 2011;144:29–35.

89. Zabdrodsky M, Calabrese L, Tosoni A, et al. Major surgery in elderly head and neck cancer patients: immediate and long-term surgical results and complication rates. Surg Oncol 2004;13:249–55.

90. Lacouurreye O, Brasnu D, Perie S, et al. Supracricoid partial laryngectomies in the elderly: mortality, complications and functional outcome. Laryngoscope 1998;108: 237–42.

91. Shestak KC, Jones NF, Wu W, et al. Effect of advanced age and medical disease on the outcome of microvascular reconstruction for head and neck defects. Head Neck 1992;14:14–8.

92. Bridger AG, O'Brien CJ, Lee KK. Advanced patient age should not preclude the use of free-flap reconstruction for head and neck cancer. Am J Surg 1994;168:425–8.

93. Malata CM, Cooter RD, Batchelor AG, et al. Microvascular free-tissue transfers in elderly patients: the Leeds experience. Plast Reconstr Surg 1996;98:1234–41.

94. Shaari CM, Buchbinder D, Costantino PD, et al. Complications of microvascular head and neck surgery in the elderly. Arch Otolaryngol Head Neck Surg 1998;124:407–11.

95. Pompei S, Tedesco M, Pozzi M, et al. Age as a risk factor in cervicofacial reconstruction. J Exp Clin Cancer Res 1998;18:209–12.

96. Moorthy SS, Radpour S. Management of anesthesia in geriatric patients undergoing head and neck surgery. Ear Nose Throat J 1999;78:496–8.

97. Fu KK, Pajak TF, Trotti A, et al. A Radiation Therapy Oncology Group (RTOG phase III randomized study to compare hyperfractionation and two variants of accelerated fractionation to standard fractionation radiotherapy for head and neck squamous cell carcinomas: first report of RTOG 9003. Int J Radiat Oncol Biol Phys 2000;48:7–16.

98. Nguyen LN, Ang KK. Radiotherapy for cancer of the head and neck: altered fractionation regimens. Lancet Oncol 2002;3:693–701.

99. Bourhis J, Overgaard J, Audry H, et al. Meta-Analysis of Radiotherapy in Carcinomas of Head and neck (MARCH) Collaborative Group. Hyperfractionated or accelerated radiotherapy in head and neck cancer: a meta-analysis. Lancet 2006;368:843–54.

100. Zachariah B, Balducci L, Venkattaramanabaji GV, et al. Radiotherapy for cancer patients aged 80 and older: a study of effectiveness and side-effects. Int J Radiat Oncol Biol Phys 1997;39:1125–9.

101. Mitsuhashi N, Hayakawa K, Yamakawa M, et al. Cancer in patients aged 90 years or older: radiation therapy. Radiology 1999;211:829–33.

102. Schofield CP, Sykes AJ, Slevin NJ, et al. Radiotherapy for head and neck cancer in elderly patients. Radiother Oncol 2003;69:34–7.

103. Oguchi M, Ikeda H, Watanabe T, et al. Experiences of 23 patients > or = 90 years of age treated with radiation therapy. Int J Radiat Oncol Biol Phys 1998;41:407–13.

104. Agiris A, Li Y, Murphy BA, et al. Outcome of elderly patients with recurrent or metastatic head and neck cancer treated with cisplatin-based chemotherapy. J Clin Oncol 2004;22:262–8.

105. Takeda J, Tanaka T, Koufuji K, et al. Gastric cancer surgery in patients aged at least 80 years old. Hepatogastroenterology 1994;41:516–20.

106. Audisio RA, Veronesi P, Ferrario L, et al. Elective surgery of gastrointestinal tumours in the aged. Ann Oncol 1997;8:317–27.

107. Gretschel S, Estevez-Schwarz L, Hünerbein M, et al. Gastric cancer surgery in elderly patients. World J Surg 2006;30:1468–74.

108. Conglio A, Tiberio GA, Busti M, et al. Surgical treatment for gastric carcinoma in the elderly. J Surg Oncol 2004;88:201–5.

109. Pisanu A, Montisci A, Piu A, et al. Curative surgery for gastric cancer in the elderly: treatment decisions, surgical morbidity, mortality, prognosis and quality of life. Tumouri 2007;93:478–84.

110. Bittner R, Butters M, Ulrich M, et al. Total gastrectomy: updated operative mortality and long-term survival with particular reference to patients older than 70 years of age. Ann Surg 1996;224:37–42.

111. Otsuji E, Fujiyama J, Takagi T, et al. Results of total gastrectomy with extended lymphade-nectomy for gastric cancer in elderly patients. J Surg Oncol 2005;91:232–6.

112. Benchimol D, Le Goff D, Fotiadis C, et al. La chirurgie d'éxerèse du cancer de l'estomac après 75 ans. Chirurgie 1989;115:436–45.

113. Eguchi T, Fujii M, Takayama T. Mortality for gastric cancer in elderly patients. J Surg Oncol 2003;84:132–6.

114. Hoffman KE, Neville BA, Memon HJ, et al. Adjuvant therapy for elderly patients with resected gastric adenocarcinoma: population-based practices and treatment effec-tiveness. Cancer 2011. [Epub ahead of print].

115. Choi JY, Shim KN, Roh SH, et al. Clinicopathological characteristics of gastric cancer and survival improvement by surgical treatment in the elderly. Korean J Gastroenterol 2011;58:9–19.

116. Cho GS, Kim W, Kim HH, et al. Multicentre study of the safety of laparoscopic subtotal gastrectomy for gastric cancer in the elderly. Br J Surg 2009;96:1437–42.

117. Sun Y, Yang Y. Study for the quality of life following total gastrectomy of gastric carcinoma. Hepatogastroenterology 2011;58:669–73.

118. Stein HJ, Sendler A, Siewert JR. Site-dependent resection techniques for gastric cancer. Surg Oncol Clin N Am 2002;11:405–14.

119. Memon MA, Subramanya MS, Khan S, et al. Meta-analysis of D1 versus D2 gastrectomy for gastric adenocarcinoma. Ann Surg 2011;253:900–11.

120. Wu AW, Xu GW, Wang HY, et al. Neoadjuvant chemotherapy versus none for resectable gastric cancer. Cochrane Database Syst Rev 2007;4:CD005047.

121. Saif MW, Makrilla N, Zalonis A, et al. Gastric cancer in the elderly: an overview. Eur J Surg Oncol 2010;36:709–17.

122. Cijs TM, Verhoef C, Steyerberg EW, et al. Outcome of esophagectomy for cancer in elderly patients. Ann Thorac Surg 2010;90:900–7.

123. Jougon JB, Ballester M, Duffy J, et al. Esophagectomy for cancer in the patient aged 70 years and older. Ann Thorac Surg 1997;63:1423–7.

124. Alexiou C, Beggs D, Salama FD, et al. Surgery for esophageal cancer in elderly patients: the view from Nottingham. J Thorac Cardiovasc Surg 1998;116:545–53.

125. Sabel MS, Smith JL, Nava HR, et al. Esophageal resection for carcinoma in patients older than 70 years. Ann Surg Oncol 2002;9:210–4.

126. Bonavina L, Incarbone R, Saino G, et al. Clinical outcome and survival after esophagectomy for carcinoma in elderly patients. Dis Esophagus 2003;16:90–3.

127. Ruol A, Portale G, Zaninotto G, et al. Results of esophagectomy for esophageal cancer in elderly patients: age has little influence on outcome and survival. J Thorac Cardiovasc Surg 2007;133:1186–92.

128. Ruol A, Portale G, Castoro C, et al. Effects of neoadjuvant therapy on perioperative morbidity in elderly patients undergoing esophagectomy for esophageal cancer. Ann Surg Oncol 2007;14:3243–50.

129. Shimada H, Shiratori T, Okazumi S, et al. Surgical outcome of elderly patients 75 years of age and older with thoracic esophageal carcinoma. World J Surg 2007;31:773–9.

130. Morita M, Egashira A, Yoshida R, et al. Esophagectomy in patients 80 years of age and older with carcinoma of the thoracic esophagus. J Gastroenterol 2008;43:345–51.

131. Takeno S, Takahashi Y, Watanabe S, et al. Esophagectomy in patients aged over 80 years with esophageal cancer. Hepatogastroenterology 2008;55:453–6.

132. Nakui M, Chino O, Ozawa S. Treatment of esophageal cancer in elderly patients. Gan To Kagaku Ryoho 2010;37:2813–6.

133. Elsayed H, Whittle I, McShane J, et al. The influence of age on mortality and survival in patients undergoing oesophagogastrectomies. A seven-year experience in a tertiary centre. Interact Cardiovasc Thorac Surg 2010;11:65–9.

134. Yang HX, Ling L, Zhang X, et al. Outcome of elderly patients with oesophageal squamous cell carcinoma after surgery. Br J Surg 2010;97:862–7.
135. Zehetner J, Lipham JC, Ayazi S, et al. Esophagectomy for cancer in octogenarians. Dis Esophagus 2010;23:666–9.
136. Fogh SE, Yu A, Kubicek GJ, et al. Do elderly patients experience increased perioperative or postoperative morbidity or mortality when given neoadjuvant chemoradiation before esophagectomy? Int J Radiat Oncol Biol Phys 2011;80:1372–6.
137. Tekkis PP, Poloniecki JD, Thompson MR, et al. ACPGBI Colorectal Cancer Study 2002: part A – unadjusted outcomes. Part B – risk adjusted outcomes. The ACPGBI Colorectal Cancer Model. Available at: http://www.acpgbi.org.uk. Access September 15, 2011.
138. Colorectal Cancer Collaborative Group. Surgery for colorectal cancer in elderly patients. Lancet 2000;356:968–74.
139. Koperna T, Kisser M, Schulz F. Emergency surgery for colon cancer in the aged. Arch Surg1997;132:1032–7.
140. Ficorella C, Cannita K, Ricevuto E. The adjuvant therapy of colonic carcinoma in old age. Minerva Med 1999;90:232–3.
141. Pavlidis TE, Marakis G, Ballas K, et al. Safety of bowel resection for colorectal surgical emergency in the elderly. Colorectal Dis 2006;8:657–62.
142. Law WL, Choi HK, Chu KW. Comparison of stenting with emergency surgery as palliative treatment for obstructing primary left-sided colorectal cancer. Br J Surg 2003;90:1429–33.
143. Ng KC, Law WL, Lee YM, et al. Self expanding metallic stents as a bridge to surgery versus emergency resection for obstructing left sided colorectal cancer: A case-matched study. J Gastrointest Surg 2006;10:798–803.
144. Carne PW, Frye JN, Robertson GM, et al. Stents or open operation for palliation of colorectal cancer: a retrospective, cohort study of perioperative outcome and long-term survival. Dis Colon Rectum 2004;47:1455–61.
145. van Hooft JE, Fockens P, Marinelli AW, et al. Premature closure of the Dutch Stent-in I study. Lancet 2006;368:1573–4.
146. Audisio RA, Zbar AP, Johnson FE. Clinical trials for colonic stents. Lancet 2007; 369(9557):188–9.
147. Targownik LE, Spiegel BM, Sack J, et al. Colonic stent vs. emergency surgery for management of acute left-sided malignant colonic obstruction: a decision analysis. Gastrointest Endosc 2004;60:865–74.
148. Guo MG, Feng Y, Zheng Q, et al. Comparison of self-expanding metal stents and urgent surgery for left-sided malignant colonic obstruction in elderly patients. Dig Dis Sci 2011;56:2706–10.
149. Selinger CP, Ramesh J, Martin DF. Long-term success of colonic stent insertion is influenced by indication but not by length of stent or site of obstruction. Int J Colorectal Dis 2011;26:215–8.
150. Trompetas V, Saunders M, Gossage J, et al. Shortcomings in colonic stenting to palliate large bowel obstruction from extracolonic malignancies. Int J Colorectal Dis 2010;25:851–4.
151. Chautard J, Alves A, Zalinski S, et al. Laparoscopic colorectal surgery in elderly patients: a matched case-control study in 178 patients. J Am Coll Surg 2008;206:255–60.
152. Pinto RA, Ruiz D, Edden Y, et al. How reliable is laparoscopic colorectal surgery compared with laparotomy for octogenarians? Surg Endosc 2011;25:2692–8.
153. Fiscon V, Portale G, Migliorini G, et al. Laparoscopic resection of colorectal cancer in elderly patients. Tumori 2010;96:704–8.
154. Robinson CN, Balentine CJ, Marshall CL, et al. Minimally invasive surgery improves short-term outcomes in elderly colorectal cancer patients. J Surg Res 2011;166:182–8.

155. Verheijen PM, Stevenson AR, Lumley JW, et al. Laparoscopic resection of advanced colorectal cancer. Br J Surg 2011;98:427–30.

156. Nozaki I, Kubo Y, Kurita A, et al. Laparoscopic colectomy for colorectal cancer patients with previous abdominal surgery. Hepatogastroenterology 2008;55:943–6.

157. Casillas S, Delaney CP, Senagore AJ, et al. Does conversion of a laparoscopic colectomy adversely affect patient outcome? Dis Colon Rectum 2004;47:1680–5.

158. Shankar A, Taylor I. Treatment of colorectal cancer in patients aged over 75. Eur J Surg Oncol 1998;24:391–5.

159. Catena F, Pasqualini E, Tonini V, et al. Emergency surgery of colorectal cancer in patients older than 80 years of age. Ann Ital Chir 2002;73:173–80.

160. Au HJ, Mulder KE, Fields AL. Systematic review of management of colorectal cancer in elderly patients. Clin Colorectal Cancer 2003;3:165–71.

161. Fietkau R, Zettl H, Klöcking S, et al. Incidence, therapy and prognosis of colorectal cancer in different age groups. A population-based cohort study of the Rostock Cancer Registry. Strahlenther Onkol 2004;180:478–87.

162. Chiappa A, Zbar AP, Bertani E, et al. Surgical treatment of advanced colorectal cancer in the elderly. Chir Ital 2005;57:589–96.

163. Richter P, Milanowski W, Bucki K, et al. Age as a prognostic factor in colorectal cancer treatment. Przegl Lek 2005;62:1440–3.

164. Heriot AG, Tekkis PP, Smith JJ, et al. Prediction of postoperative mortality in elderly patients with colorectal cancer. Dis Colon Rectum 2006;49:816–24.

165. Isobe H, Takasu N, Mizutani M, et al. Management of colorectal cancer in elderly patients over 80 years old. Nippon Ronen Igakkai Zasshi 2007;44:599–605.

166. Basili G, Lorenzetti L, Biondi G, et al. Colorectal cancer in the elderly. Is there a role for safe and curative surgery? ANZ J Surg 2008;78:466–70.

167. Aparicio T, Navazesh A, Boutron I, et al. Half of elderly patients routinely treated for colorectal cancer receive a sub-standard treatment. Crit Rev Oncol Hematol 2009; 71:249–57.

168. Matasar MJ, Sundararajan V, Grann VR, et al. Management of colorectal cancer in elderly patients: focus on the cost of chemotherapy. Drugs Aging 2004;21:113–33.

169. Chiappa A, Bertani E, Zbar AP, et al. Surgery for advanced colorectal cancer in elderly patients with special emphasis for radio-chemotherapy role. Hepatogastroenterology 2007;54:740–5.

170. Bouvier AM, Jooste V, Bonnetain F, et al. Adjuvant treatments do not alter the quality of life in elderly patients with colorectal cancer: a population-based study. Cancer 2008;113:879–86.

171. Pasetto LM, Friso ML, Pucciarelli S, et al. Rectal cancer neoadjuvant treatment in elderly patients. Anticancer Res 2006;26:3913–23.

172. Mantello G, Berardi R, Cardinali M, et al. Feasibility of preoperative chemoradiation in rectal cancer patients aged 70 and older. J Exp Clin Cancer Res 2005;24:541–6.

173. Hotta T, Takifuji K, Yokoyama S, et al. Rectal cancer surgery in the elderly: analysis of consecutive 158 patients with stage III rectal cancer. Langenbecks Arch Surg 2007;392:549–58.

174. Lorchel F, Peignaux K, Créhange G, et al. Preoperative radiotherapy in elderly patients with rectal cancer. Gastroenterol Clin Biol 2007;31:436–41.

175. Fiorica F, Cartei F, Carau B, et al. Adjuvant radiotherapy on older and oldest elderly rectal cancer patients. Arch Gerontol Geriatr 2009;49:54–9.

176. Reddy N, Yu J, Fakih MG. Toxicities and survival among octogenarians and nonagenarians with colorectal cancer treated with chemotherapy or concurrent chemoradiation therapy. Clin Colorectal Cancer 2007;6:362–6.

177. Agostini M, Pasetto LM, Pucciarelli S, et al. Glutathione S-transferase P1 Ile105Val polymorphism is associated with haematological toxicity in elderly rectal cancer patients receiving preoperative chemoradiotherapy. Drugs Aging 2008;25:531–9.

178. Habr-Gama A, Perez RO, Proscurshim I, et al. Patterns of failure and survival for nonoperative treatment of stage c0 distal rectal cancer following neoadjuvant chemoradiation therapy. J Gastrointest Surg 2006;10:1319–28.

179. Bege T, Lelong B, Esterni B, et al. The learning curve for the laparoscopic approach to conservative mesorectal excision for rectal cancer: lessons drawn from a single institution's experience. Ann Surg 2010;251:249–53.

180. Del Rio P, Dell'Abate P, Gomes B, et al. Analysis of risk factors for complications in 262 cases of laparoscopic colectomy. Ann Ital Chir 2010;81:21–30.

181. Akiyoshi T, Kuroyanagi H, Oya M, et al. Short-term outcomes of laparoscopic rectal surgery for primary rectal cancer in elderly patients: is it safe and beneficial? J Gastrointest Surg 2009;13:1614–8.

182. Ogiso S, Yamaguchi T, Hata H, et al. Evaluation of factors affecting the difficulty of laparoscopic anterior resection for rectal cancer: "narrow pelvis" is not a contraindication. Surg Endosc 2011;25:1907–12.

183. de Campos-Lobato LF, Alves-Ferreira PC, Geisler DP, et al. Benefits of laparoscopy: does the disease condition that indicated colectomy matter? Am Surg 2011;77:527–33.

184. Brown CJ, Raval MJ. Advances in minimally invasive surgery in the treatment of colorectal cancer. Expert Rev Anticancer Ther 2008;8:111–23.

185. Kurian A, Suryadevara S, Ramaraju D, et al. In-hospital and 6-month mortality rates after open elective vs open emergent colectomy in patients older than 80 years. Dis Colon Rectum 2011;54:467–71.

186. Marks JH, Kawun UB, Hamdan W, et al. Redefining contraindications to laparoscopic colorectal resection for high-risk patients. Surg Endosc 2008;22:1899–904.

187. Frasson M, Braga M, Vignali A, et al. Benefits of laparoscopic colorectal resection are more pronounced in elderly patients. Dis Colon Rectum 2008;51:296–300.

188. Blair SL, Schwarz RE. Advanced age does not contribute to increased risks or poor outcome after major abdominal operations. Am Surg 2001;67:1123–7.

189. Monson K, Litvak DA, Bold RJ. Surgery in the aged population: surgical oncology. Arch Surg 2003;138:1061–7.

190. Evers BM, Townsend CM Jr, Thompson JC. Organ physiology of aging. Surg Clin North Am 1994;74:23–39.

191. Webb TP, Duthie E Jr. Geriatrics for surgeons: infusing life into an aging subject. J Surg Educ 2008;65:91–4.

192. Van Leeuwen BL, Kristjansson SR, Audisio RA. Should specialized oncogeriatric surgeons operate older unfit cancer patients? Eur J Surg Oncol 2010;36:S18–22.

193. Cheema FN, Abraham NS, Berger DH, et al. Novel approaches to perioperative assessment and intervention may improve long-term outcomes after colorectal cancer resection in older adults. Ann Surg 2011;253:867–74.

Early Breast Cancer in the Older Woman

Ari VanderWalde, MD, MPH[a],*, Arti Hurria, MD[b]

KEYWORDS

- Breast cancer • Geriatric • Surgery • Radiation therapy
- Chemotherapy • Targeted therapy
- Supportive care oncology

Breast cancer, like many common cancers, is primarily a disease of older adults. In the United States the median age at the diagnosis of breast cancer is 61 years, and 41% of breast cancers are diagnosed in women aged 65 or older.[1] The median age at death from breast cancer is 68 years, and 57% of deaths from breast cancer occur in those aged 65 and older.[1] Early stage breast cancer in the older adult, as in the younger adult, is a curable disease in the overwhelming majority of patients. Almost 1.5 million women over age 65 in the United States are breast cancer survivors, and over 820,000 of these women are aged 75 or older.[1]

Breast cancer incidence and mortality increases with age (**Table 1**). Older adults are both more likely to develop breast cancer than younger adults and significantly more likely to die of breast cancer. For example, the oldest women (age 85+) have approximately three times the incidence of breast cancer compared with the youngest population (age 40–44), and they have 13 times the mortality rate.[2] In this article the authors review the data regarding breast cancer in the older adult and discuss tumor biology, treatment modalities, and the short-term and long-term risks and benefits of therapy in the older adult.

BREAST CANCER BIOLOGY IN THE OLDER WOMAN

There are conflicting data regarding whether there are true differences in breast cancer biology with increasing age. Some evidence suggests that the biology of breast cancer in older adults is less aggressive.[3–6] A review of Surveillance

Disclosures: Dr VanderWalde is a full-time employee of Amgen and owns stock in Amgen. Dr Hurria's research has been supported by NIH research grants K23 AG026749 and U13 AG038151. She has received additional research funding from Celgene and GlaxoSmithKline and has also served as a consultant to Amgen and Genentech.
[a] Global Development-Oncology, Amgen Inc, One Amgen Center Drive, MS 38-B-A, Thousand Oaks, California 91320, USA
[b] Department of Medical Oncology, City of Hope Comprehensive Cancer Center, 1500 East Duarte Road, Duarte, California 91010, USA
* Corresponding author.
E-mail address: ariv@amgen.com

Table 1		
Incidence and mortality of female breast cancer by age in the United States 1995–2007		
Age	Incidence (per 100,000 person-years)	Mortality (per 100,000 person-years)
40–44	121	14
45–49	186	23
50–54	226	35
55–59	280	49
60–64	349	62
65–69	394	73
70–74	410	87
75–79	434	108
80–84	422	134
85+	339	177

Data from Altekruse S, Kosary C, Krapcho M, et al. SEER cancer statistics review, 1975–2007. National Cancer Institute. Available at: http://seer.cancer.gov/csr/1975_2007/</csr/1975_2007/>.

Epidemiology End Results (SEER) and San Antonio databases demonstrated that older women are more likely to have hormone receptor–positive and HER2-negative disease, which generally carries a more favorable prognosis.[7] On the other hand, there is also evidence to support the hypothesis that breast cancer is more aggressive in older adults. For example, one study showed up to 19% of older women to have luminal B tumors, which are more likely to present with higher grade, larger size, and increased propensity to spread to lymph nodes, despite being hormone receptor–positive.[8]

Despite the conflicting data regarding breast cancer biology and aging, there are sound data suggesting that the specific characteristics of the tumor should be used to guide the risk of relapse and the need for therapy. For example, Oncotype DX (Genomic Health) is a 21-gene assay that yields a score that predicts both breast cancer recurrence and chemotherapy efficacy. Among 668 patients with node-negative breast cancer treated with tamoxifen, Oncotype DX accurately predicted whether there was a low, intermediate, or high risk of distant recurrence and was also predictive of overall survival. The gene signature's predictive effect was ultimately independent of age.[9]

TREATMENT PATTERNS IN OLDER ADULTS WITH BREAST CANCER

There are ample data suggesting a difference in treatment patterns between older and younger adults with breast cancer. There are several possible reasons for these differences including other comorbidities (outweighing the risk of cancer or influencing treatment tolerance), poorer perceived or actual treatment tolerance,[10] poorer access to care, and/or patient or physician preference.[10–16] The challenge that faces older adults and their physicians is that there are less evidence-based data to guide these decisions in older adults secondary to the underenrollment of older adults in clinical trials.[17–22] For example, a review of Southwest Oncology Group therapeutic trials revealed that in studies of breast cancer, only 9% of women enrolled were aged 65 or older, despite the fact that 49% of the population of women with breast cancer were in this age group.[17] Patients over 70 made up only 20% of subjects enrolled in US Food and Drug Administration registration trials from 1995 to 1999, although they made up fully 46% of the US cancer population in that period.[18] Underenrollment of older patients with breast cancer contributes to a poorer understanding of the risks and benefits associated with cancer treatment and might be a contributing factor in the difference in treatment patterns in this population. However, recent studies focusing specifically on older patients have successfully reached their target accrual, demonstrating the feasibility of studying this population of patients and successfully accruing to clinical trials that guide key clinical questions.[23,24]

TREATMENT

Treatment for breast cancer is multimodal in nature. Patients with early breast cancer are generally treated with surgery with or without radiation therapy for local control of the disease. Treatment options for the control of systemic disease include chemotherapy, endocrine therapy (for hormone receptor–positive disease), and trastuzumab (for HER2-positive disease). Each of these modalities of therapy has specific risks and benefits as related to the older patient, and each is discussed in turn.

Surgery

Surgical treatment options for breast cancer generally include mastectomy or breast conserving surgery (BCS, also known as lumpectomy), with sentinel lymph node sampling and axillary lymph node dissection if the sentinel node reveals tumor. However, it is unclear whether older women receive surgery as often as younger adults and whether they receive similar modalities of surgery. One study demonstrated that older women are less likely to receive BCS (as compared with mastectomy or no surgical treatment), with only 21% of adults aged 80 or older receiving this modality.[25] Single-institution studies suggest that older women have comparable rates of receiving definitive surgery to younger adults.[26,27] One institution reported that 95% of women age 70 or older received primary surgery and 89% received axillary lymph node dissection as appropriate.[27]

It is recognized that age is not the most important factor in the determination of surgical risk.[28,29] The Preoperative Assessment of Cancer in the Elderly (PACE)[29–33] incorporates elements of the comprehensive geriatric assessment (CGA), a brief fatigue inventory, performance status measures, and the American Society of Anesthesiologists grade.[31] In a prospective international study, 460 consecutive older adults with cancer underwent PACE prior to surgery. Poor performance status, dependence in instrumental activities of daily living, and moderate to severe fatigue were found to be independently associated with an extended hospital stay in the postoperative period.[32] Another recent trial demonstrated that measures of frailty, disability, and comorbidity are good predictors of 6-month postoperative mortality or institutionalization after major surgery in older adults.[34] However, even at the extremes of age, breast cancer surgery carries a low risk of morbidity and mortality and can be done under local anesthesia with sedation if the risk of general anesthesia is too great.[35]

Other investigators have evaluated whether it is necessary to perform surgery for breast cancer in older adults, particularly if there is an alternative treatment option such as an antiestrogen. The data from individual studies are conflicting. A Cochrane Review[36] reported on seven trials of women aged 70 or older that randomized women to surgery with or without tamoxifen as compared with tamoxifen alone (without surgery). The women were all considered to be fit for general anesthesia and surgery. Nevertheless, despite improved progression-free survival among women treated with surgery as compared with those treated with tamoxifen alone, there was no benefit seen in overall survival.[36] The impact of cancer progression on overall quality of life remains a consideration.

The role of axillary lymph node dissection is an area of active study. A randomized study of 473 women with hormone receptor–positive early breast cancer compared surgery with axillary dissection versus surgery alone in women over age 60 with clinically node-negative disease. The median age was 74 years, and all women received tamoxifen following surgery. At a median follow-up of 6.6 years, both disease-free survival and overall survival were similar in the two groups. (Hazard ratio [HR] for disease-free survival, 1.06; 95% confidence interval [CI], 0.79–1.42; $P = .69$; HR for overall survival, 1.05; 95% CI, 0.76–1.46; $P = .77$). The investigators concluded that it is possible to avoid axillary dissection in women aged 60 or older with hormone receptor–positive early breast cancer and clinically node-negative disease, provided that the patients receive endocrine therapy following surgery.[37]

An interesting dilemma exists for prevention of future cancer, specifically among those older patients who would like to reduce their risk of developing future breast cancer by prophylactic removal of the breasts. In older women with a personal history of breast cancer, the benefit of prophylactic surgery is uncertain. In a large retrospective cohort study of women diagnosed with unilateral breast cancer between 1979 and 1999, it was found that of 1072 women who had a prophylactic contralateral mastectomy following their first cancer only 0.5% developed a contralateral breast cancer as compared with 2.7% of those who underwent surveillance alone. (HR 0.03, 95% CI 0.006–0.13).[38] Although the risk of developing contralateral breast cancer increased with age, this difference was not statistically significant (HR age ≥70 vs age ≤39 5.3, 95% CI 0.4–73). As such, making a conclusion about the relative efficacy of contralateral prophylactic mastectomy in older adults as compared with younger adults is difficult.[38]

Additionally, any overall survival benefit achieved by prophylactic surgery for breast cancer has been shown to be minimal to nonexistent.[38,39] A recent analysis found that the relative cost-effectiveness of prophylactic mastectomy decreases with increasing age, to the point that the investigators conclude that it is not cost-effective to perform prophylactic mastectomies in patients with a first diagnosis at age70 or older because fewer quality-adjusted life years are gained by prophylactic surgery in the older cohort than in the younger.[40] Even in women with a genetic mutation that predisposes to development of future breast and ovarian cancers (such as BRCA-1 and 2), prophylactic mastectomy and oophorectomy may not be of significant benefit in older women. A decision analysis by Schrag and colleagues[41] revealed that in women with a first breast cancer diagnosis at age 60 or older, the gains in life expectancy from contralateral mastectomy and bilateral oophorectomy are modest at best and range from 2 weeks in low-penetrance mutations to 1.1 years in high-penetrance mutations.[41]

Radiation Therapy

In the general population of women with early breast cancer, radiation treatment to the preserved breast is standard practice following BCS.[42] When combined with whole-breast radiation, BCS has equivalent survival compared with mastectomy alone. Additionally, it is standard to administer radiation to the chest wall following mastectomy if the tumor size is greater than 5 cm or if there are four or more positive lymph nodes.[43] Radiation is used as an adjunct to surgery and decreases the risk of both local recurrence and subsequent metastatic spread.

In older women, studies have shown that whole-breast radiation given per guidelines following surgery decreases in-breast recurrences, and some studies suggest that it lengthens disease-specific and overall survival as well. Use of radiation, however, decreases with increasing age. Truong and colleagues[44] reported on 4836 patients aged 50 to 89 with early stage breast cancer who were treated with BCS, of whom 773 were older than 74 years. After a median follow-up of 7.5 years, radiation omission was associated with significantly increased relapse rates as well as poorer disease-specific and all-cause survival. As many as 26% of women over age 74 did not receive radiation compared with only 7% of those aged 50 to 64.[44] In women aged 50 or older with small, node-negative breast cancer, radiation, when added to tamoxifen following BCS, has been shown to significantly decrease the risk of breast or axillary recurrence compared with tamoxifen alone.[45] A randomized trial evaluated the benefits of radiation following breast conserving therapy in women aged 70 and older with stage I hormone receptor–positive breast cancer who received systemic therapy with tamoxifen. After a median of 5 years of follow-up, receipt of radiation decreased the rate of local or regional recurrence from 4% to 1%; however, there was no difference in overall survival, and the majority of patients who died succumbed to comorbid diseases other than breast cancer.[23]

A recent update of these data seems to confirm a lack of survival benefit of radiation even after 10.5 years follow-up, although the risk of local recurrence remained higher in the tamoxifen-only group (9% in tamoxifen only arm vs 2% in tamoxifen plus radiation, $P = .0001$).[46] A retrospective analysis of the SEER-Medicare database evaluated the efficacy of radiation in women aged 70 or older in the treatment of small node-negative cancer. A 4% absolute lower risk of second ipsilateral breast cancer (in-breast recurrence) was seen in the cohort who received radiation. Women aged 70 to 79 with few comorbidities benefited most, whereas women aged 80 or older or those with significant comorbidities were less likely to benefit.[47]

On the other hand, patients with high-risk breast cancer, even after mastectomy, seem to clearly benefit from radiation. Using a SEER database review, Smith and colleagues[48] identified 11,594 women aged 70 or older who received mastectomy for breast cancer and classified them as either low-risk, intermediate-risk, or high-risk based on tumor size and lymph node involvement. The investigators then looked to see whether receipt of postmastectomy radiation therapy improved survival in women with high-risk disease (defined as tumor over 5 cm and/or four or more positive lymph nodes). After a median follow-up of 6.2 years, radiation therapy was associated with a significant improvement in overall survival (HR 0.85, $P = .02$). There was no corresponding improvement seen among low-risk or intermediate-risk patients.[48]

Radiation therapy seems to be relatively well-tolerated in older adults,[46,49] although unique issues that might identify those older women as less likely to tolerate radiation include poor functional status, preexisting pulmonary or cardiac disease, and decreased cognition.[50] Additionally, shorter courses of radiation, such as single-dose intraoperative radiotherapy, are under study and show promise in preventing in-breast recurrences in a subset of patients with early breast cancer with possibly fewer long-term side effects.[51]

Systemic Therapy

Various types of systemic therapy are used in early breast cancer, including endocrine therapy, cytotoxic chemotherapy, targeted therapy with trastuzumab, or various combinations of these. A list of agents commonly used in the adjuvant setting in early breast cancer is provided in **Table 2**.

Table 2	
Systemic therapies commonly used in early breast cancer	
Chemotherapy	Cyclophosphamide
	Doxorubicin
	Epirubicin
	Paclitaxel
	Docetaxel
	Fluorouracil (5-FU)
	Methotrexate
	Carboplatin
Endocrine Therapy	Tamoxifen
	Letrozole
	Anastrazole
	Exemestane
Targeted Therapy	Trastuzumab

Endocrine therapy

Women with hormone receptor–positive breast cancer benefit from adjuvant endocrine therapy following surgery and/or radiation for early breast cancer, both in improved relapse-free and overall survival. The two classes of endocrine therapy available in the postsurgical setting for postmenopausal women are the selective estrogen receptor modulator (tamoxifen) and the aromatase inhibitors (AIs).

Both tamoxifen and AIs have been shown across age groups of postmenopausal women with hormone receptor–positive disease to lower the risk of relapse and increase overall survival.[52] Five years of tamoxifen has been shown to decrease the annual rate of breast cancer recurrence by 51%, and this benefit is preserved regardless of patient age.[52] Therapy with an AI is only beneficial in postmenopausal women. Randomized studies in the adjuvant setting of AIs verses tamoxifen demonstrate that AIs are associated with an improvement in disease-free survival; however, there is no difference in overall survival.[53,54] As such, it is generally recommended that older adults with hormone receptor–positive disease (the overwhelming majority of cases) be treated with AIs; however, the optimal strategy of using AIs (ie, whether to use AIs alone or in sequence following tamoxifen) remains unclear, and the risks and benefits of each drug need to be considered for the individual patient.[55] Treatment with tamoxifen is associated with an increased risk of endometrial cancer and thromboembolism. On the other hand, tamoxifen has a beneficial effect on bone health in older women and improves the lipid profile. AIs do not increase the risk of endometrial cancer; however, they do carry a risk of thromboembolism (although this risk is lower in comparison with tamoxifen). In addition, treatment with AIs is associated with a loss in bone mineral density.[56–59] Attention to maximizing bone health is important in all older adults; however, it is particularly important in women receiving therapy with an AI.

Although tamoxifen and AIs are both generally well-tolerated in the older adult, their efficacy may be hindered by nonadherence or discontinuation of endocrine therapy.[60] One study reported the observation that adults over age 65 are 28% less likely to be adherent to endocrine therapy than younger adults.[61] However, studies are conflicting, and whereas some suggest age is a risk factor,[60,61] others do not.[62,63] Regardless, rates of discontinuation of endocrine therapy are higher than might be expected in survivors of early breast cancer,[63,64] and as such, it remains important to determine which older adults are likely to benefit from endocrine therapy and which are more likely to develop intolerable side effects. During therapy, asking about medication usage is essential, and if adverse effects prevent adherence, consideration should be given to switching agents. Because endocrine therapy is oral, it is also important to ensure that the patient is able to manage her own medications or has someone to help manage them on her behalf.

Chemotherapy

The decision of when and whether to offer adjuvant chemotherapy to a woman with early breast cancer is one of the more difficult clinical decisions in the field, regardless of the age of the patient. Chemotherapy in early breast cancer may be given prior to surgery (neoadjuvant) or after surgery (adjuvant). The purpose of neoadjuvant or adjuvant chemotherapy is to decrease the risk of relapse and mortality from breast cancer by treating micrometastatic disease. A randomized study demonstrated equivalent efficacy in terms of relapse-free and overall survival, whether the chemotherapy is given in a neoadjuvant or adjuvant fashion.[65] Neoadjuvant therapy may also serve to decrease tumor size in order to enable the option of breast conservation.

The decision of whether or not to administer chemotherapy is based on weighing the tumor characteristics (risk of relapse and mortality), the patient characteristics (such as functional status, comorbidity, social support, risk of toxicities), and the patient's preferences. Tools such as Oncotype DX, a 21-gene panel assay, can be used among patients with node-negative hormone receptor–positive disease to predict the risk of relapse as well as the efficacy of adjuvant chemotherapy.[9]

Data from the Early Breast Cancer Trialists' Collaborative Group suggest a decreasing benefit from adjuvant chemotherapy with increasing age; however, the investigators acknowledge that too few women over the age of 70 were included in randomized clinical trials to reliably inform these data.[66] In contrast, a metaanalysis of patients enrolled in randomized clinical trials for node-positive disease demonstrated that older women seem to derive similar benefit from the experimental chemotherapy arm as younger individuals.[67]

Prospective randomized clinical trials have demonstrated a benefit to standard adjuvant chemotherapy in an older adult. The Cancer and Leukemia Group B Study 49907 randomized women aged 65 or older with early breast cancer to receive either standard chemotherapy (doxorubicin and cyclophosphamide [AC] or cyclophosphamide, methotrexate, and 5-fluorouracil [CMF]) or capecitabine, an oral chemotherapeutic agent not routinely given as a single agent for the adjuvant treatment of breast cancer. Treatment with capecitabine was associated with a significantly worse relapse-free survival, with women receiving capecitabine more than twice as likely to relapse as those receiving standard chemotherapy. Additionally, a statistically significant overall survival benefit was seen with standard chemotherapy (HR 1.85, 95% CI 1.11–3.08). Rates of clinically significant adverse events were similar across study arms, with a slight increase in the rate of febrile neutropenia in the standard chemotherapy arm as compared with capecitabine (8%–9% vs 1%).[24] Rates of adherence to capecitabine (an oral agent) were 75% and were not related to age.[68] Another prospective randomized controlled trial has been reported that randomized women older than age 65 with early breast cancer to either tamoxifen alone or tamoxifen combined with six cycles of chemotherapy.[69] The investigators found that a statistically significant decreased risk of relapse after 6 years of follow-up with the chemotherapy group (HR of relapse in tamoxifen alone arm 1.93, 95% CI 1.70–2.17). Older adults also did not seem to exhibit unacceptable levels of toxicity with the chemotherapy regimen given.

Other studies have been geared toward developing therapeutic strategies to avoid exposure to anthracyclines, which are associated with a risk of cardiac toxicity. A randomized clinical trial in the general population of early breast cancer demonstrated that a taxane-containing regimen (docetaxel + cyclophosphamide for four cycles [TC]), was superior to a standard anthracycline-based regimen (AC for four cycles) in both disease-free and overall survival, even among the older adults in the study.[70] Toxicity was similar across age groups, although older women had more febrile neutropenia with TC and more anemia with AC.

In summary, adjuvant chemotherapy when indicated should not be withheld from older women with early breast cancer because of age alone, and chemotherapeutic agent choice can be similar to that which would be used in the younger adult.[71] However, the clinician must be particularly attuned to potential toxicities and should develop an individualized plan with the patient to determine the likelihood of benefit given other risk factors.

Toxicity considerations with chemotherapy in the older woman with breast cancer

Supportive care, given together with chemotherapy, is of primary importance among older adults, who have increased risk of both bone marrow suppression and gastrointestinal toxicity from cytotoxic agents. Older adults with breast cancer are at a higher risk of neutropenia with chemotherapy. In a study of adults aged 65 and older with lung, breast, or ovarian carcinoma or non-Hodgkin lymphoma, patients were randomized to receive prophylactic pegfilgrastim (Neulasta; Amgen) before every cycle of various chemotherapeutic regimens, or secondary pegfilgrastim administered only at the discretion of the treating physician. Median age was 72 years. Of the 686 patients with solid tumors analyzed, the rate of grade 4 neutropenia was 54% (95% CI 53%–64%) in those who received growth factor by physician discretion and only 22% (95% CI 18%–27%) in those who received growth factor after every cycle. The prevalence of febrile neutropenia was 10% in the physician discretion arm but only 4% in the every-cycle arm ($P = .001$). Patients who received pegfilgrastim after every cycle were significantly less likely to experience dose delays or dose reductions or to receive antibiotics. The investigators concluded that growth factors should be used proactively in all older adults to support the optimal delivery of chemotherapy.[72]

Because of the risk of neutropenic infections among older adults, multiple consensus panels including the National Comprehensive Cancer Network, the American Society of Clinical Oncology, the European Organization for Research and Treatment of Cancer, and the International Society of Geriatric Oncology, have recommended up-front prophylactic granulocyte-colony stimulating factor in any older adult treated with chemotherapy regimens with febrile neutropenia rates comparable to those seen with the CHOP regimen (cyclophosphamide, vincristine, doxorubicin, and prednisone) given for non-Hodgkin lymphoma.[73]

Although it has been thought that older patients experience less chemotherapy-induced nausea and vomiting than younger patients, this remains a potentially serious complication. Older adults tend to have decreased nutritional reserve and fluid stores, and thus periods of prolonged nausea or vomiting can quickly lead to dehydration, electrolyte imbalances, and malnutrition. The combination of doxorubicin and cyclophosphamide, commonly used in adjuvant therapy, is in particular highly emetogenic, whereas the agents are at least moderately emetogenic when given alone.[74] Therefore, it is important to anticipate moderate to severe nausea and vomiting in older adults receiving adjuvant chemotherapy for breast cancer,[75] to deliver adequate prophylactic antinausea medication,[76] and to have a low threshold to initiate further treatment for symptoms.[73] Additionally, older adults are more likely to develop diarrhea, dehydration, and mucositis with chemotherapy than younger adults[77] and are less likely to tolerate these complications than younger adults.[73] Therefore early treatment of the symptoms, including intravenous fluid, should be delivered to older adults with a low threshold for hospitalization if needed.[73]

Predicting chemotherapy toxicity in older adults with cancer

Investigators have sought to determine whether items in a CGA, in combination with those captured in daily clinical practice, can identify patients at risk for chemotherapy toxicity. A multiinstitutional prospective study of 500 patients with cancer identified the following factors predictive of chemotherapy toxicity: (1) age 73 or older, (2) cancer type (gastrointestinal or genitourinary), (3) receipt of polychemotherapy, (4) receipt of standard dosing of chemotherapy, (5) creatinine clearance greater than 34 ml/min (Jelliffe formula using ideal weight), (6) hemoglobin (male: <11 g/dL, female: <10 g/dL), (7) the need for assistance with taking medications, (8) one or more falls in the last 6 months, (9) hearing impairment, (10) limited in walking one block, and (11) decreased social activities due to physical or emotional health.[78] The Chemotherapy Risk Assessment Scale for High-Age Patients (CRASH) study evaluated 562 patients with cancer and found that albumin, need for assistance with instrumental activities of daily living, lactate dehydrogenase, and diastolic blood pressure were predictive of hematologic toxicity and hemoglobin, creatinine clearance, albumin, self-rated health, comorbidity, electrocortico-graphy performance status, mini-mental status examination, and mini-nutritional assessment were predictive of nonhematologic toxicity.[79]

Trastuzumab

Approximately 25% of breast cancers overexpress the HER2 receptor on the surface of tumor cells, making those cancers potentially susceptible to HER2-directed therapy.[80] Whereas many anti-HER2 agents are being studied in early breast cancer, the only agent currently widely approved or used in this setting is trastuzumab (Herceptin; Roche), a monoclonal antibody that prevents dimerization of HER2 and has been shown to increase disease-free and overall survival in early breast cancer when given in combination with chemotherapy.[81,82] Older age has been shown to correlate with increased likelihood of developing therapy-related cardiotoxicity, however, and this risk is compounded when trastuzumab is given with an anthracy-cline-containing regimen.[83,84] Additionally, baseline cardiac comorbidities such as diabetes or preexisting coronary artery disease may predispose to higher rates of trastuzumab-related cardiotoxicity in older adults.[85]

Single-agent trastuzumab has a relatively favorable side effect profile; however, trastuzumab given in combination with chemotherapy is associated with increased toxicities in older adults. An ongoing trial known as RESPECT is randomizing women aged 70 to 80 with HER2-positive early breast cancer to therapy with either trastuzumab alone or trastuzumab with standard chemotherapy.[86] This trial may guide clinicians in the future to determine whether older women with early stage HER2-positive breast cancer who receive trastuzumab can safely forgo adjuvant chemotherapy and the associated toxicities.

FOLLOW-UP OF THE OLDER WOMAN WITH BREAST CANCER
Long-Term Side Effects in the Older Adult

Constitutional side effects

Fatigue is one of the most pervasive side effects of breast cancer treatment, may occur in up to 80% to 90% of patients treated,[87] and is the most commonly described side effect in women who undergo chemotherapy for breast cancer.[88] However, being a subjective symptom, it is notoriously difficult to measure and as such may often be neglected.[89] Cancer-related fatigue differs from normal fatigue in that it is more insidious in onset, more pervasive, and more severe.[90] Breast cancer survivors often continue to experience fatigue well after the completion of treatment. Experience of fatigue seems to be the case regardless of the modality of treatment used, although the percentage may be somewhat higher in those who received both radiation and chemotherapy than in either group alone.[91] Because of the effect on functioning, fatigue can be debilitating in older adults, who may have limited mobility, energy, or functioning at baseline. Fatigue could potentially be the difference between an active, functioning older adult and a bed-bound dependent one. Broekel and colleagues[92] surveyed 61 women with a history of breast cancer who had completed adjuvant chemotherapy an average of 18 months previously and compared their self-reports of fatigue to 59 women with no history of cancer. The investigators found that women with a history of cancer reported an average level of fatigue 50% greater than the controls and were more likely to report that fatigue interfered with their overall quality of life, their ability to work, and their concentration.[92] Although it has been postulated that older patients with cancer may have more severe fatigue than younger patients with cancer, definitive evidence for this is lacking.[89]

Whereas there are few studies comparing rates of fatigue in older adults to younger adults, one study demonstrated that age-related factors tend to play a larger role than cancer-related factors in older long-term survivors of cancer.[93] Yoga, nutritional therapy, and sleep therapy have been shown to decrease fatigue in survivors.[89,94] Various exercise programs have been associated with decreased fatigue and improved quality of life in patients with breast cancer.[89,95] Evaluation and treatment of comorbid conditions including depression and anemia may help to decrease contributing factors associated with fatigue. It is particularly important to evaluate for and treat depression in older adults, because depression is commonly missed in routine evaluation.

The term *chemobrain* has been used to describe the subjective cognitive effects of chemotherapy. However, this entity is complex, is likely multifactorial, and impacts a subset of the population who receive therapy.[96] It has been noted that patient report of neurocognitive impairment often does not correlate with neurocognitive impairment on performance tests.[96–98] Older adults may also be vulnerable to neurocognitive changes associated with cancer therapy. One study among older adults who received chemotherapy for breast cancer showed a significant decline in cognitive function, at least in the short term, although the differences in degree of cognitive decline were not compared with the nongeriatric adult population.[96] A more recent study found that age and baseline cognitive reserve seem to be associated with rates of cognitive changes with chemotherapy, although these changes begin to improve over time, and it is not clear what the impact of these changes are on functioning.[99] Further research is needed to identify the magnitude of the problem, the risk factors for cognitive decline, and interventions to help minimize this risk.

Cardiac side effects

Anthracyclines (doxorubicin, daunorubicin, epirubicin) can be associated with a dose-dependent progressive decrease in systolic left ventricular ejection fraction, indistinguishable from coronary heart disease due to other causes. The cardiomyopathy can also present as symptomatic or asymptomatic diastolic dysfunction.[100] Age at the time of treatment is also a risk factor. One study showed that adults over the age of 65 who received anthracycline-containing chemotherapy for breast cancer had an HR for developing cardiomyopathy of 2.48 (95% CI, 2.10–2.93) compared with the nonchemotherapy group. Likewise, the HR was 1.38 (95% CI, 1.25–1.52) for overt congestive heart failure.[101] Using the SEER database, Pinder and colleagues[102] found that women between the ages of 66 and 70 treated with anthracyclines for breast cancer had an HR of 1.26 (95% CI, 1.12–1.42) for developing cardiomyopathy compared with those who had not received anthracyclines. However, the relationship was not linear. In women aged 71 to 80, there was no association between chemotherapy type and cardiomyopathy.[102]

Trastuzumab is also associated with cardiomyopathy, especially when given in conjunction with an anthracycline. In the National Surgical Adjuvant Breast and Bowel Project B-31, cardiac events were measured among patients receiving AC followed in sequence by trastuzumab and paclitaxel. The cumulative incidence of symptomatic heart failure at 3 years was 4.1% in the trastuzumab group compared with 0.8% in the nontrastuzumab group. No cardiac deaths were reported in the trastuzumab group. Increasing age and decreasing ejection fraction after AC and before starting trastuzumab were independent risk factors for developing congestive heart failure.[83]

Skeletal side effects

Older adults with bone loss are more likely to have increased risks of falling, fracture, disability, and even mortality. AIs are potent inhibitors of estradiol production and hence markedly decrease circulating levels of estrogen.[103] The depletion of estrogen has a negative effect on bone density.[103–105] A number of phase III clinical trials reporting on the adjuvant use of AIs have reported increased risk of bone loss and osteoporotic fracture in patients taking AIs as compared with those taking either tamoxifen or not on therapy.[56–59,106–113]

Calcium, vitamin D, and weight-bearing exercise strengthen bones and decrease the risk of development of osteoporosis. Effective screening strategies and treatment should be used in older adults at risk for treatment related bone loss. The American Society of Clinical Oncology has recommended for all women with breast cancer over the age of 65 to have annual dual-energy x-ray absorptiometry scans of the spine and hip and to take calcium and vitamin D supplements. If the osteoporosis threshold (T score ≤ -2.5) is reached, addition of a bisphosphonate is recommended.[114] For patients with osteopenia, the decision to use bisphosphonates should be individualized.

INTEGRATING GERIATRIC PRINCIPLES INTO ONCOLOGY TREATMENT DECISIONS

An integral part of the cancer treatment decision is to determine whether the patient will die of cancer, or simply with cancer. Furthermore, one needs to weigh whether the cancer is likely to cause significant disability for the patient in his/her lifetime.[115] Whereas younger patients with breast cancer can usually anticipate that having a diagnosis of cancer will shorten their life expectancy without treatment, the same may not be true for older adults. The prevalence of comorbid conditions increases with age.[116,117] Competing comorbidities increase the risk that the older adult with cancer may die of another cause.[118] In this setting, an indolent cancer may not influence the life span or quality of life of the patient.

However, estimating life expectancy is a complex process that extends beyond chronological age. Tools and prognostic indices developed and reported in the geriatric literature can help assist oncologists in estimating life expectancy. Walter and Covinsky,[119] using US life table data, described life expectancy by upper, middle, and lower quartiles. For example, although the median additional life expectancy for a 70-year-old woman is 15.7 years, 25% of 70-year-old women can expect to live an additional 21.3 years or more, whereas 25% of these women can only expect an additional 9.5 years or less.[119] Carey and colleagues[120] developed a functional morbidity index that takes into account age, gender, and self-reported functional status to stratify adults aged 70 or older into varying risk groups for 2-year mortality. Lee and colleagues[121] developed a similar tool for clinicians to determine 4-year mortality. This tool takes into account comorbid conditions as well as age, gender, and functional status. Estimation of life expectancy may have significant intraobserver variability, and these tools could help to more precisely fine-tune our estimates.

A CGA has been used in the general geriatric population to assist in an evaluation of life expectancy, to identify vulnerable older adults, and to guide interventions to optimize care in this population.[122–124] The domains evaluated in a CGA include functional status, comorbidity, cognitive function, psychological state, social support, nutritional status, and a review of concurrent medications. Consensus guidelines recommend the routine use of the CGA for older adults with cancer; however, the exact means of integrating a CGA into oncology practice is an area of active research.[125,126] It has been postulated that the CGA might be used to guide treatment strategies in older adults with cancer,[124,127,128] and various cancer-specific geriatric assessments have been proposed.[128,129] In addition, researchers are using the CGA to identify factors predictive of chemotherapy toxicity risk[78,79] as well as nomograms for overall survival.[130] The majority of this research has been performed among patients with all cancer types; however, specific studies focusing on the treatment of older adults with breast cancer is under way.

SUMMARY

Care of the older woman with early breast cancer is of particular importance to both the oncologist and geriatrician because of both the prevalence of the disease in this population as well as the subtleties necessary in individualizing treatment decisions. In general, older women are able to tolerate many of the same modalities of treatment for early breast cancer as younger women, but special consideration must be given to future life expectancy, comorbidities, and other elements that might be identified using a CGA. Both short-term and long-term side effects of cancer therapies can be clinically important in the older woman, and appropriate screening and support for these toxicities are necessary.

REFERENCES

1. Howlader N, Noone A, Krapcho M, et al, editors. SEER cancer statistics review, 1975–2008. National Cancer Institute. Available at: http://seer.cancer.gov/csr/1975_2008/. Accessed September 15, 2011.
2. Altekruse S, Kosary C, Krapcho M, et al. SEER cancer statistics review, 1975–2007. National Cancer Institute. Available at: http://seer.cancer.gov/csr/1975_2007/</csr/1975_2007/>. Accessed September 15, 2011.
3. Balducci L. Geriatric oncology. Crit Rev Oncol Hematol 2003;46:211–20.
4. Balducci L, Beghe C. Cancer and age in the USA. Crit Rev Oncol Hematol 2001;37:137–45.
5. Audisio RA, Bozzetti F, Gennari R, et al. The surgical management of elderly cancer patients; recommendations of the SIOG surgical task force. Eur J Cancer 2004;40:926–38.
6. Gennari R, Curigliano G, Rotmensz N, et al. Breast carcinoma in elderly women: features of disease presentation, choice of local and systemic treatments compared with younger postmenopausal patients. Cancer 2004;101:1302–10.
7. Diab SG, Elledge RM, Clark GM. Tumor characteristics and clinical outcome of elderly women with breast cancer. J Natl Cancer Inst 2000;92:550–6.

8. Durbecq V, Ameye L, Veys I, et al. A significant proportion of elderly patients develop hormone-dependent "luminal-B" tumours associated with aggressive characteristics. Crit Rev Oncol Hematol 2008;67:80–92.

9. Paik S, Shak S, Tang G, et al. A multigene assay to predict recurrence of tamoxifen-treated, node-negative breast cancer. N Engl J Med 2004;351:2817–26.

10. Lichtman SM, Wildiers H, Chatelut E, et al. International Society of Geriatric Oncology Chemotherapy Taskforce: evaluation of chemotherapy in older patients–an analysis of the medical literature. J Clin Oncol 2007;25:1832–43.

11. Droz JP, Aapro M, Balducci L. Overcoming challenges associated with chemotherapy treatment in the senior adult population. Crit Rev Oncol Hematol 2008; 68(Suppl 1):S1–8.

12. Extermann M, Albrand G, Chen H, et al. Are older French patients as willing as older American patients to undertake chemotherapy? J Clin Oncol 2003;21:3214–9.

13. DeMichele A, Putt M, Zhang Y, et al. Older age predicts a decline in adjuvant chemotherapy recommendations for patients with breast carcinoma: evidence from a tertiary care cohort of chemotherapy-eligible patients. Cancer 2003;97:2150–9.

14. Shariat SF, Sfakianos JP, Droller MJ, et al. The effect of age and gender on bladder cancer: a critical review of the literature. BJU Int 2009;105:300–8.

15. Hall WH, Jani AB, Ryu JK, et al. The impact of age and comorbidity on survival outcomes and treatment patterns in prostate cancer. Prostate Cancer Prostatic Dis 2005;8:22–30.

16. Lane BR, Abouassaly R, Gao T, et al. Active treatment of localized renal tumors may not impact overall survival in patients aged 75 years or older. Cancer 2010;116: 3119–26.

17. Hutchins LF, Unger JM, Crowley JJ, et al. Underrepresentation of patients 65 years of age or older in cancer-treatment trials. N Engl J Med 1999;341:2061–7.

18. Talarico L, Chen G, Pazdur R. Enrollment of elderly patients in clinical trials for cancer drug registration: a 7-year experience by the US Food and Drug Administration. J Clin Oncol 2004;22:4626–31.

19. Yee KW, Pater JL, Pho L, et al. Enrollment of older patients in cancer treatment trials in Canada: why is age a barrier? J Clin Oncol 2003;21:1618–23.

20. Murthy VH, Krumholz HM, Gross CP. Participation in cancer clinical trials: race-, sex-, and age-based disparities. JAMA 2004;291:2720–6.

21. Stewart JH, Bertoni AG, Staten JL, et al. Participation in surgical oncology clinical trials: gender-, race/ethnicity-, and age-based disparities. Ann Surg Oncol 2007;14: 3328–34.

22. Lewis JH, Kilgore ML, Goldman DP, et al. Participation of patients 65 years of age or older in cancer clinical trials. J Clin Oncol 2003;21:1383–9.

23. Hughes KS, Schnaper LA, Berry D, et al. Lumpectomy plus tamoxifen with or without irradiation in women 70 years of age or older with early breast cancer. N Engl J Med 2004;351:971–7.

24. Muss HB, Berry DA, Cirrincione CT, et al. Adjuvant chemotherapy in older women with early-stage breast cancer. N Engl J Med 2009;360:2055–65.

25. Bouchardy C, Rapiti E, Fioretta G, et al. Undertreatment strongly decreases prognosis of breast cancer in elderly women. J Clin Oncol 2003;21:3580–7.

26. Rosenkranz KM, Bedrosian I, Feng L, et al. Breast cancer in the very elderly: treatment patterns and complications in a tertiary cancer center. Am J Surg 2006; 192:541–4.

27. Laki F, Kirova Y, Savignoni A, et al. Management of operable invasive breast cancer in women over the age of 70: long term results of a large-scale single-institution experience. Ann Surg Oncol 2010;17:1530–8.

28. Kemeny MM, Busch-Devereaux E, Merriam LT, et al. Cancer surgery in the elderly. Hematol Oncol Clin North Am 2000;14:169–92.

29. Ramesh HS, Pope D, Gennari R, et al. Optimising surgical management of elderly cancer patients. World J Surg Oncol 2005;3:17.

30. Audisio RA, Ramesh H, Longo WE, et al. Preoperative assessment of surgical risk in oncogeriatric patients. Oncologist 2005;10:262–8.

31. Pope D, Ramesh H, Gennari R, et al. Pre-operative assessment of cancer in the elderly (PACE): a comprehensive assessment of underlying characteristics of elderly cancer patients prior to elective surgery. Surg Oncol 2006;15:189–97.

32. Audisio RA, Pope D, Ramesh HS, et al. Shall we operate? Preoperative assessment in elderly cancer patients (PACE) can help. A SIOG surgical task force prospective study. Crit Rev Oncol Hematol 2008;65:156–63.

33. Ramesh HS, Jain S, Audisio RA. Implications of aging in surgical oncology. Cancer J 2005;11:488–94.

34. Bremmer MA, Beekman AT, Deeg DJ, et al. Inflammatory markers in late-life depression: results from a population-based study. J Affect Disord 2008;106:249–55.

35. Reed M, Audisio R, Wyld L. The role of surgery in the treatment of older women with breast cancer. Clin Oncol (R Coll Radiol) 2009;21:103–10.

36. Hind D, Wyld L, Reed MW. Surgery, with or without tamoxifen, vs tamoxifen alone for older women with operable breast cancer: Cochrane review. Br J Cancer 2007;96:1025–9.

37. International Breast Cancer Study Group, Rudenstam CM, Zahrieh D, et al. Randomized trial comparing axillary clearance versus no axillary clearance in older patients with breast cancer: first results of International Breast Cancer Study Group Trial 10-93. J Clin Oncol 2006;24:337–44.

38. Herrinton LJ, Barlow WE, Yu O, et al. Efficacy of prophylactic mastectomy in women with unilateral breast cancer: a cancer research network project. J Clin Oncol 2005;23:4275–86.

39. Lostumbo L, Carbine N, Wallace J, et al. Prophylactic mastectomy for the prevention of breast cancer. Cochrane Database Syst Rev 2004;4:CD002748.

40. Zendejas B, Moriarty J, O'Byrne J, et al. Cost-effectiveness of contralateral prophylactic mastectomy versus routine surveillance in patients with unilateral breast cancer. J Clin Oncol 2011;29:2993–3000.

41. Schrag D, Kuntz KM, Garber JE, et al. Life expectancy gains from cancer prevention strategies for women with breast cancer and BRCA1 or BRCA2 mutations. JAMA 2000;283:617–24.

42. Fisher B, Anderseon S, Bryant J, et al. Twenty-year follow-up of a randomized trial comparing total mastectomy, lumpectomy, and lumpectomy plus irradiation for the treatment of invasive breast cancer. N Engl J Med 2002;347:1233–41.

43. Jagsi R, Pierce L. Postmastectomy radiation therapy for patients with locally advanced breast cancer. Semin Radiat Oncol 2009;19:236–43.

44. Truong PT, Bernstein V, Lesperance M, et al. Radiotherapy omission after breast-conserving surgery is associated with reduced breast cancer-specific survival in elderly women with breast cancer. Am J Surg 2006;191:749–55.

45. Fyles AW, McCready DR, Manchul LA, et al. Tamoxifen with or without breast irradiation in women 50 years of age or older with early breast cancer. N Engl J Med 2004;351:963–70.

46. Hughes KS, Schnaper LA, Cirrincione C, et al. Lumpectomy plus tamoxifen with or without irradiation in women age 70 or older with early breast cancer [abstract]. J Clin Oncol 2010;28(15 Suppl):507.

47. Smith BD, Gross CP, Smith GL, et al. Effectiveness of radiation therapy for older women with early breast cancer. J Natl Cancer Inst 2006;98:681–90.

48. Smith BD, Haffty BG, Hurria A, et al. Postmastectomy radiation and survival in older women with breast cancer. J Clin Oncol 2006;24:4901–7.
49. Wyckoff J, Greenberg H, Sanderson R, et al. Breast irradiation in the older woman: a toxicity study. J Am Geriatr Soc 1994;42:150–2.
50. Albrand G, Terret C. Early breast cancer in the elderly: assessment and management considerations. Drugs Aging 2008;25:35–45.
51. Vaidya JS, Joseph DJ, Tobias JS, et al. Targeted intraoperative radiotherapy versus whole breast radiotherapy for breast cancer (TARGIT-A trial): an international, prospective, randomised, non-inferiority phase 3 trial. Lancet 2010;376:91–102.
52. Early Breast Cancer Trialists' Collaborative Group (EBCTCG). Effects of chemotherapy and hormonal therapy for early breast cancer on recurrence and 15-year survival. Lancet 2005;365:1687–717.
53. Cuzick J, Sestak I, Baum M, et al. Effect of anastrazole and tamoxifen as adjuvant treatment for early-stage breast cancer: 10-year analysis of the ATAC trial. Lancet Oncol 2010;11:1135–41.
54. Thurlimann B, Keshaviah A, Coates AS, et al. A comparison of letrozole and tamoxifen in postmenopausal women with early breast cancer. N Engl J Med 2005;353:2747–57.
55. Gandhi S, Verma S. Early breast cancer in the older woman. Oncologist 2011;16: 479–85.
56. Coleman RE, Banks LM, Girgis SI, et al. Skeletal effects of exemestane on bone-mineral density, bone biomarkers, and fracture incidence in postmenopausal women with early breast cancer participating in the Intergroup Exemestane Study (IES): a randomised controlled study. Lancet Oncol 2007;8:119–27.
57. Eastell R, Adams JE, Coleman RE, et al. Effect of anastrozole on bone mineral density: 5-year results from the anastrozole, tamoxifen, alone or in combination trial 18233230. J Clin Oncol 2008;26:1051–7.
58. Lonning PE, Geisler J, Krag LE, et al. Effects of exemestane administered for 2 years versus placebo on bone mineral density, bone biomarkers, and plasma lipids in patients with surgically resected early breast cancer. J Clin Oncol 2005;23:5126–37.
59. Perez EA, Josse RG, Pritchard KI, et al. Effect of letrozole versus placebo on bone mineral density in women with primary breast cancer completing 5 or more years of adjuvant tamoxifen: a companion study to NCIC CTG MA.17. J Clin Oncol 2006;24: 3629–35.
60. van Herk-Sukel MP, van de Poll-Franse LV, Voogd AC, et al. Half of breast cancer patients discontinue tamoxifen and any endocrine treatment before the end of the recommended treatment period of 5 years: a population-based analysis. Breast Cancer Res Treat 2010;122:843–51.
61. Hershman DL, Kushi LH, Shao T, et al. Early discontinuation and nonadherence to adjuvant hormonal therapy in a cohort of 8,769 early-stage breast cancer patients. J Clin Oncol 2010;28:4120–8.
62. Ziller V, Kalder M, Albert US, et al. Adherence to adjuvant endocrine therapy in postmenopausal women with breast cancer. Ann Oncol 2009;20:431–6.
63. Partridge AH, Wang PS, Winer EP, et al. Nonadherence to adjuvant tamoxifen therapy in women with primary breast cancer. J Clin Oncol 2003;21:602–6.
64. Partridge AH, LaFountain A, Mayer E, et al. Adherence to initial adjuvant anastrozole therapy among women with early-stage breast cancer. J Clin Oncol 2008;26: 556–62.
65. Rastogi P, Anderson SJ, Bear HD, et al. Preoperative chemotherapy: updates of National Surgical Adjuvant Breast and Bowel Project Protocols B-18 and B-27. J Clin Oncol 2008;26:778–85.

66. Effects of chemotherapy and hormonal therapy for early breast cancer on recurrence and 15-year survival: an overview of the randomised trials. Lancet 2005;365:1687–717.

67. Muss HB, Woolf S, Berry D, et al. Adjuvant chemotherapy in older and younger women with lymph node-positive breast cancer. JAMA 2005;293:1073–81.

68. Partridge AH, Archer L, Kornblith AB, et al. Adherence and persistence with oral adjuvant chemotherapy in older women with early-stage breast cancer in CALGB 49907: adherence companion study 60104. J Clin Oncol 2010;28:2418–22.

69. Fargeot P, Bonneterre J, Roche H, et al. Disease-free survival advantage of weekly epirubicin plus tamoxifen versus tamoxifen alone as adjuvant treatment of operable, node-positive, elderly breast cancer patients: 6-year follow-up results of the French Adjuvant Study Group 08 trial. J Clin Oncol 2004;22:4674–82.

70. Jones S, Holmes FA, O'Shaughnessy J, et al. Docetaxel with cyclophosphamide is associated with an overall survival benefit compared with doxorubicin and cyclophosphamide: 7-year follow-up of USA Oncology Research Trial 9735. J Clin Oncol 2009;27:1177–83.

71. Wildiers H, Kunkler I, Biganzoli L, et al. Management of breast cancer in elderly individuals: recommendations of the International Society of Geriatric Oncology. Lancet Oncol 2007;8:1101–15.

72. Balducci L, Al-Halawani H, Charu V, et al. Elderly cancer patients receiving chemotherapy benefit from first-cycle pegfilgrastim. Oncologist 2007;12:1416–24.

73. Pallis AG, Fortpied C, Wedding U, et al. EORTC elderly task force position paper: approach to the older cancer patient. Eur J Cancer 2010;46:1502–13.

74. NCCN Clinical practice guidelines in oncology. Antiemesis, V.1.2012. Available at: http://www.nccn.org/professionals/physician_gls/PDF/antiemesis.pdf. Accessed September 1, 2011.

75. Gridelli C. Same old story? Do we need to modify our supportive care treatment of elderly cancer patients? Focus on antiemetics. Drugs Aging 2004;21:825–32.

76. Aapro M, Johnson J. Chemotherapy-induced emesis in elderly cancer patients: the role of $5-HT_3$-receptor antagonists in the first 24 hours. Gerontology 2005;51:287–96.

77. Baker SD, Grochow LB. Pharmacology of cancer chemotherapy in the older person. Clin Geriatr Med 1997;13:169–83.

78. Hurria A, Togawa K, Mohile SG, et al. Predicting chemotherapy toxicity in older adults with cancer: a prospective multicenter study. J Clin Oncol 2011;29:3457–65.

79. Extermann M, Boler I, Reich R, et al. The chemotherapy risk assessment scale for high-age patients (CRASH) score: design and validation [abstract]. J Clin Oncol 2010;28:(Suppl 15):9000.

80. Slamon DJ, Godolphin W, Jones LA, et al. Studies of the HER-2/neu proto-oncogene in human breast and ovarian cancer. Science 1989;244:707–12.

81. Perez EA, Romond EH, Suman VJ, et al. Four-year follow-up of trastuzumab plus adjuvant chemotherapy for operable human epidermal growth factor receptor 2-positive breast cancer: joint analysis of data from NCCTG N9831 and NSABP B-31. J Clin Oncol 2011;29:3366–73.

82. Gianni L, Dafni U, Gelber RD, et al. Treatment with trastuzumab for 1 year after adjuvant chemotherapy in patients with HER2-positive early breast cancer: a 4-year follow-up of a randomised controlled trial. Lancet Oncol 2011;12:236–44.

83. Tan-Chiu E, Yothers G, Romond E, et al. Assessment of cardiac dysfunction in a randomized trial comparing doxorubicin and cyclophosphamide followed by paclitaxel, with or without trastuzumab as adjuvant therapy in node-positive, human epidermal growth factor receptor 2-overexpressing breast cancer: NSABP B-31. J Clin Oncol 2005;23:7811–9.

84. Perez EA, Suman VJ, Davidson NE, et al. Cardiac safety analysis of doxorubicin and cyclophosphamide followed by paclitaxel with or without trastuzumab in the North Central Cancer Treatment Group N9831 adjuvant breast cancer trial. J Clin Oncol 2008;26:1231–8.

85. Serrano C, Cortes J, De Mattos-Arruda L, et al. Trastuzumab-related cardiotoxicity in the elderly: a role for cardiovascular risk factors. Ann Oncol 2011. [Epub ahead of print].

86. Sawaki M, Tokudome N, Mizuno T, et al. Evaluation of trastuzumab without chemotherapy as a post-operative adjuvant therapy in HER2-positive elderly breast cancer patients: randomized controlled trial [RESPECT (N-SAS BC07)]. Jpn J Clin Oncol 2011;41:709–12.

87. Lawrence DP, Kupelnick B, Miller K, et al. Evidence report on the occurrence, assessment, and treatment of fatigue in cancer patients. J Natl Cancer Inst Monogr 2004:40–50.

88. de Jong N, Candel MJ, Schouten HC, et al. Prevalence and course of fatigue in breast cancer patients receiving adjuvant chemotherapy. Ann Oncol 2004;15:896–905.

89. Rao AV, Cohen HJ. Fatigue in older cancer patients: etiology, assessment, and treatment. Semin Oncol 2008;35:633–42.

90. Davis MP, Khoshknabi D, Yue GH. Management of fatigue in cancer patients. Curr Pain Headache Rep 2006;10:260–9.

91. Bower JE, Ganz PA, Desmond KA, et al. Fatigue in long-term breast carcinoma survivors: a longitudinal investigation. Cancer 2006;106:751–8.

92. Broekel JA Jacobsen PB, Horton J, et al. Characteristics and correlates of fatigue after adjuvant chemotherapy for breast cancer. J Clin Oncol 1998;16:1689–96.

93. Deimling GT, Bowman KF, Wagner LJ. The effects of cancer-related pain and fatigue on functioning of older adult, long-term cancer survivors. Cancer Nurs 2007;30:421–33.

94. Bower JE, Woolery A, Sternlieb B, et al. Yoga for cancer patients and survivors. Cancer Control 2005;12:165–71.

95. Peddle CJ, Au HJ, Courneya KS. Associations between exercise, quality of life, and fatigue in colorectal cancer survivors. Dis Colon Rectum 2008;51:1242–8.

96. Hurria A, Rosen C, Hudis C, et al. Cognitive function of older patients receiving adjuvant chemotherapy for breast cancer: a pilot prospective longitudinal study. J Am Geriatr Soc 2006;54:925–31.

97. Ahles TA, Saykin AJ, Furstenberg CT, et al. Quality of life of long-term survivors of breast cancer and lymphoma treated with standard-dose chemotherapy or local therapy. J Clin Oncol 2005;23:4399–405.

98. Schagen SB, van Dam FS, Muller MJ, et al. Cognitive deficits after postoperative adjuvant chemotherapy for breast carcinoma. Cancer 1999;85:640–50.

99. Ahles TA, Saykin AJ, McDonald BC, et al. Longitudinal assessment of cognitive changes associated with adjuvant treatment for breast cancer: impact of age and cognitive reserve. J Clin Oncol 2010;28:4434–40.

100. Carver JR, Shapiro CL, Ng A, et al. American Society of Clinical Oncology clinical evidence review on the ongoing care of adult cancer survivors: cardiac and pulmonary late effects. J Clin Oncol 2007;25:3991–4008.

101. Doyle JJ, Neugut AI, Jacobson JS, et al. Chemotherapy and cardiotoxicity in older breast cancer patients: a population-based study. J Clin Oncol 2005;23:8597–605.

102. Pinder M, Duane Z, Goodwin, JS, et al. Congestive heart failure in older women treated with adjuvant anthracycline chemotherapy for breast cancer. J Clin Oncol 2007;25:3794–6.

103. Reid DM, Doughty J, Eastell R, et al. Guidance for the management of breast cancer treatment-induced bone loss: A consensus position statement from a UK Expert Group. Cancer Treat Rev 2008;34:S3–S18.

104. Saad F, Adachi JD, Brown JP, et al. Cancer Treatment-Induced Bone Loss in Breast and Prostate Cancer. J Clin Oncol 2008;26:5465–76.

105. Bell R, Lewis J. Assessing the risk of bone fracture among postmenopausal women who are receiving adjuvant hormonal therapy for breast cancer. Curr Med Res Opin 2007;23:1045–51.

106. Forbes J, Cuzick J, Buzdar A, et al. Effect of anastrozole and tamoxifen as adjuvant treatment for early-stage breast cancer: 100-month analysis of the ATAC trial. Lancet Oncol 2008;9:45–53.

107. Eastell R, Hannon RA, Cuzick J, et al. Effect of an aromatase inhibitor on BMD and bone turnover markers: 2-year results of the Anastrozole, Tamoxifen, Alone or in Combination (ATAC) trial (18233230). J Bone Miner Res 2006;21:1215–23.

108. Coates AS, Keshaviah A, Thurlimann B, et al. Five years of letrozole compared with tamoxifen as initial adjuvant therapy for postmenopausal women with endocrine-responsive early breast cancer: update of study BIG 1-98. J Clin Oncol 2007;25: 486–92.

109. Goss PE, Ingle JN, Martino S, et al. A randomized trial of letrozole in postmenopausal women after five years of tamoxifen therapy for early-stage breast cancer. N Engl J Med 2003;349:1793–802.

110. Geisler J, Lønning PE, Krag LE, et al. Changes in bone and lipid metabolism in postmenopausal women with early breast cancer after terminating 2-year treatment with exemestane: a randomised, placebo-controlled study. Eur J Cancer 2006;42: 2968–75.

111. Coombes RC, Kilburn LS, Snowdon CF, et al. Survival and safety of exemestane versus tamoxifen after 2-3 years' tamoxifen treatment (Intergroup Exemestane Study): a randomised controlled trial. Lancet 2007;369:559–70.

112. Hadji P, Ziller M, Kieback DG, et al. Effects of exemestane and tamoxifen on bone health within the Tamoxifen Exemestane Adjuvant Multicentre (TEAM) trial: results of a German, 12-month, prospective, randomised substudy. Ann Oncol 2009;20: 1203–9.

113. Mincey BA, Duh MS, Thomas SK, et al. Risk of cancer treatment-associated bone loss and fractures among women with breast cancer receiving aromatase inhibitors. Clin Breast Cancer 2006;7:127–32.

114. Hillner BE, Ingle JN, Chlebowski RT, et al. American Society of Clinical Oncology 2003 update on the role of bisphosphonates and bone health issues in women with breast cancer. J Clin Oncol 2003;21:4042–57.

115. Balducci L, Beghe C. Cancer in the elderly: biology, prevention, and treatment. In: Abeloff MD, Armitage JO, Niederhuber JE, et al, editors. Abeloff's clinical oncology. 4th edition. Philadelphia: Churchill Livingstone; 2008. p. 1039–49.

116. Reuben D, Rubenstein L, Hirsch S, et al. Value of functional status as a predictor of mortality: results of a prospective study. Am J Med 1992;93:663–9.

117. Extermann M, Overcash J, Lyman GH, et al. Comorbidity and functional status are independent in older cancer patients. J Clin Oncol 1998;16:1582–7.

118. Satariano WA, Ragland DR. The effect of comorbidity on 3-year survival of women with primary breast cancer. Ann Intern Med 1994;120:104–10.

119. Walter LC, Covinsky KE. Cancer screening in elderly patients: a framework for individualized decision making. JAMA 2001;285:2750–6.

120. Carey EC, Walter LC, Lindquist K, et al. Development and validation of a functional morbidity index to predict mortality in community-dwelling elders. J Gen Intern Med 2004;19:1027–33.
121. Lee SJ, Lindquist K, Segal MR, et al. Development and validation of a prognostic index for 4-year mortality in older adults. JAMA 2006;295:801–8.
122. Rao AV, Seo PH, Cohen HJ. Geriatric assessment and comorbidity. Semin Oncol 2004;31:149–59.
123. Stuck AE, Siu AL, Wieland GD, et al. Comprehensive geriatric assessment: a meta-analysis of controlled trials. Lancet 1993;342:1032–6.
124. Freyer G, Geay J, Touzet S, et al. Comprehensive geriatric assessment predicts tolerance to chemotherapy and survival in elderly patients with advanced ovarian carcinoma: a GINECO study. Ann Oncol 2005;16:1795–800.
125. Extermann M, Aapro M, Bernabei R, et al. Use of comprehensive geriatric assessment in older cancer patients: recommendations from the task force on CGA of the International Society of Geriatric Oncology (SIOG). Crit Rev Oncol Hematol 2005;55:241–52.
126. Balducci L, Cohen HJ, Engstrom PF, et al. Senior adult oncology clinical practice guidelines in oncology. J Natl Compr Canc Netw 2005;3:572–90.
127. Bernabei R, Venturiero V, Tarsitani P, et al. The comprehensive geriatric assessment: when, where, how. Crit Rev Oncol Hematol 2000;33:45–56.
128. Monfardini S, Ferrucci L, Fratino L, et al. Validation of a multidimensional evaluation scale for use in elderly cancer patients. Cancer 1996;77:395–401.
129. Hurria A, Gupta S, Zauderer M, et al. Developing a cancer-specific geriatric assessment: a feasibility study. Cancer 2005;104:1998–2005.
130. Kanesvaran R, Li H, Koo KN, et al. Analysis of prognostic factors of comprehensive geriatric assessment and development of a clinical scoring system in elderly Asian patients with cancer. J Clin Oncol 2011. [Epub ahead of print].

Ethical Dilemmas in Elderly Cancer Patients: A Perspective From the Ethics of Care

Maruscha de Vries RN, BSN[a,b,]*, Carlo J.W. Leget, PhD[c,d]

KEYWORDS
- Aging • Cancer • Treatment • Elderly • Geriatric • Ethics

Elderly cancer patients are a large and rapidly growing group of patients suffering from a range of problems including comorbidity, polypharmacy, emotional problems, functional and cognitive limitations, and a lack of social support, which require physical as well as psychosocial support. For the elderly, cancer treatment and patient experiences are far from one-size-fits-all. During the last decade, oncologists and geriatricians have begun to work together to integrate geriatric principles into oncology care. Applying geriatric principles and assessment to this older population may be helpful in decision-making by providing estimates of life expectancy, identifying vulnerability in individuals, and releasing patients' strengths, weaknesses or preferences. On the other hand, in caring for elderly cancer patients, many ethical problems can be encountered. Ethics involves more than decision-making, and in fact caring is an ethical enterprise itself. In this article an ethical approach is introduced that is especially helpful when dealing with elderly cancer patients. Two cases are discussed, first from the perspective of the traditional medical approach of principlism and subsequently from an ethics of care perspective. By adopting this latter perspective, a better view is gained of what is ethically at stake for both elderly cancer patients and their caregivers.

The authors have nothing to disclose.
[a] Division of Care and Education, Comprehensive Cancer Centre South, PO Box 231, 5600 AE, Eindhoven (IKZ), The Netherlands
[b] Program Geriatric Oncology, Netherlands (GeriOnNe), Eindhoven, The Netherlands
[c] Faculty of Humanities, Room D 242, Tilburg University, PO Box 90153, 5000 LE Tilburg, Tilburg, The Netherlands
[d] Ethics of Care, University for Humanistic Studies, Utrecht, The Netherlands
* Corresponding author. Division of Care and Education, Comprehensive Cancer Centre South, PO Box 231, 5600 AE, Eindhoven (IKZ), The Netherlands.
E-mail address: m.de.vries@ikz.nl

Clin Geriatr Med 28 (2012) 93–104
doi:10.1016/j.cger.2011.10.004
0749-0690/12/$ – see front matter © 2012 Elsevier Inc. All rights reserved.

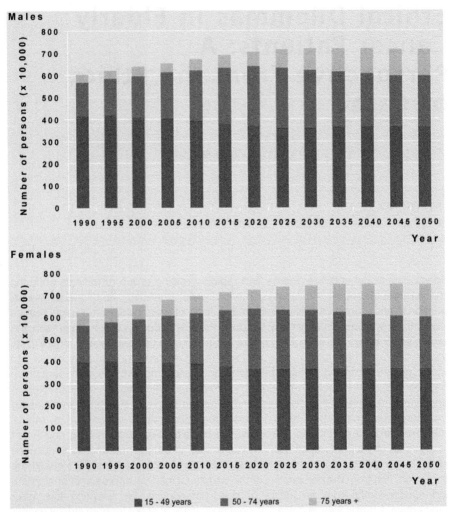

Fig. 1. Population structure from 1990 to 2050, for men and woman in various age groups. (*From* Dutch Cancer Society. Cancer in the Netherlands until 2020. Amsterdam: Dutch Cancer Society; 2011; with permission.)

AGING AND CANCER

Aging societies are facing the impact of demographic changes in the next decades. By the year 2040, 14% of the world population will be aged 65 and over, and 3.3% will be aged 80 years and over.[1]

The Netherlands faces the phenomenon of double-aging: not only are elderly people increasing in number, but they are living longer as well. The growth in numbers is among the postwar baby boomers who began to reach the age of 65 in 2010 and who will represent a sharp increase in the elderly population in The Netherlands (**Fig. 1**). The 75 and older age group will double from 7% in 2010 to 14 % in 2040.[2]

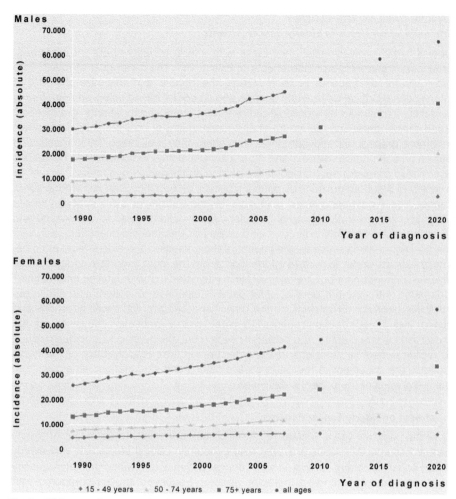

Fig. 2. All forms of cancer. Absolute incidence rates from 1989 to 2007 with projections to 2020. (*From* Dutch Cancer Society. Cancer in the Netherlands until 2020. Amsterdam: Dutch Cancer Society; 2011; with permission.)

Cancer is the first leading cause of death in the Netherlands and is frequently a disease of older individuals.[3] The absolute number of new cancer patients is projected to increase from 45,110 men and 41,690 women in 2007 to approximately 66,000 men and 57,000 women in 2020 (**Fig. 2**). This aging of the population and the fact that cancer is mainly a disease of old age will significantly increase the absolute number of cancer patients by more than 40%.

This increase will result in a substantial extra burden on society in terms of caring for cancer patients. Health services must make preparations for this increase if it is to safeguard the quality of care in the years to come.[2] As previously mentioned, medical and nursing staff in oncology for older cancer patients are confronted with a range of problems including comorbidity, polypharmacy, emotional problems, functional limitations, and a lack of social support, which require physical as well as psychosocial support.[4]

CANCER CARE IN THE ELDERLY
Communication Needs in Elderly Cancer Patients

One of health professionals' chief tasks is to inform patients about the diagnosis, prognosis, treatment, and side effects of treatment.[5] The mean goal of health care providers for all patients is to maximize the benefit and minimize the risk of interventions. Critical therapeutic choices should not be based solely on rigid, formal guidelines but should be individualized and take into account patients' preferences. Good clinical decisions require a better understanding of how patients view certain treatment procedures and outcomes that effect their well-being.[6] Communication between health care providers and older cancer patients is complicated by various age-related problems such as cognitive decline and sensory impairments, as well as a variety of other factors such as patient's beliefs, perceptions, and knowledge about cancer. Health care providers should have the knowledge and skills to communicate effectively with their older patients.[7] Older cancer patients need to understand and recall important information about their disease and treatment to deal adequately with the decision-making process, the impact of their disease, and side effects at home. These patients prefer to receive information about the most important aspects of the disease and treatment but are relatively less interested in more detailed information.[5] Compared with younger people, older patients ask fewer questions and show less proactive behavior. Physicians on the other hand, tend to ask fewer questions and spend less time communicating with older cancer patients.[7] However, at the crossroads where medical and personal needs meet, the nurse is in a unique position to facilitate medical decisions in the older person. The responsibility of the nurse includes the statement of the patient's aspirations and expectations emerging from the living word of the patient's daily life.[6]

Treatment of Elderly Cancer Patients

Over the past few years, increasing attention has been paid to treatment of elderly cancer patients. Age limits are used less frequently, clinical studies on vital elderly report equal outcomes compared with younger patients, and within the heterogeneity of elderly patients, standard therapies are less frequently applied compared with younger groups.[8] A chief characteristic of growing old is that people age at different rates. Calendar age alone is not a suitable criterion to select patients for a certain treatments.[9]

Another aspect of aging is an increased prevalence of comorbidity in general (**Fig. 3**). Cancer patients aged 70 years and older have on average three comorbidities. These comorbidities may influence risk with regard to cancer, diagnoses, evolution, and treatment. Furthermore, increased comorbidity is also associated with polypharmacy.[10]

In the elderly cancer patient, diagnostic procedures, treatment, and experiences are far from one-size-fits-all. This fact is especially true for older cancer patients, who may be more affected by certain side effects or complications of interventions. Also, these complications may have impact on mortality and the ability to return home or live independently. Premorbid patient characteristics partially determine these outcomes.[11] As a consequence, the health status of older persons cannot be evaluated by merely describing the single disease and/or by measuring the response or survival. Conversely, it is necessary to conduct a more comprehensive investigation of the functional status of the aged person after treatment.[12] Both patient and the oncologic team are doing a balancing act between potential benefits and adverse effects.

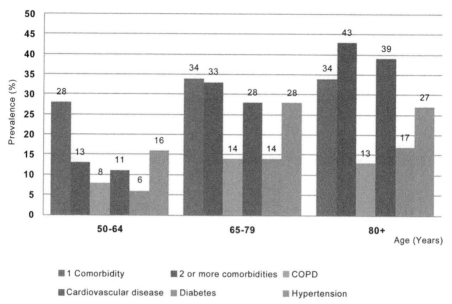

Fig. 3. Comorbidity in cancer patients-prevalence according to age. (*Courtesy of* Cancer Registry comprehensive Cancer Centre South, Eindhoven; with permission.)

Situations are even more complex for the elderly, because as a group they have other and sometimes divergent aspirations.[13,14]

Decision-Making: The Introduction of Geriatrics in Oncology Care

During the last decade, oncologists and geriatricians have begun to work together to integrate the principles of geriatrics in oncology care. The increasing use of a comprehensive geriatric assessment (CGA) is one example of this effort.[15] The CGA is a process that consists of a multidimensional data search and a process of analyzing and linking patient characteristics and creating an individualized intervention-plan carried out by a multidisciplinary team. In general the positive health care effects of CGA are established, but in oncology both CGA and the presence of geriatric syndromes still need to be implemented to tailor oncologic therapies to the needs of elderly cancer patients.[16] Applying geriatric principles and assessment to this older population may be helpful in decision-making by providing estimates of life expectancy, identifying vulnerability in individuals, and revealing patients' strengths, weaknesses, or preferences.[17] At present there are several frailty instruments to create a one-dimensional variable on vulnerability: Vulnerable Elderly Survey-13, the Edmonton Frailty scale, the Groningen Frailty Indicator, and the Tilburg Frailty Indicator.[18] At present, indices on frailty divide patients into two groups: frail and nonfrail. In treatment decisions in cancer patients, negative predictive value seems to be the most important feature of these scales, because this value allows us to select patients who can undergo standard treatment plans. This ability is important in order to avoid unnecessary loss of quality of life and enable preventive or curative interventions to be effected in good time.[19]

Nevertheless, a "go/no-go" decision in relation to the standard treatment strategy is only one of the issues in cancer care for individual patients. Professionals providing care and treatment for elderly cancer patients need to make a wide range of decisions. These decisions may relate to patients' care and treatment, but they also involve discussions with patients and families in terms of treatment and care options. These discussions can also include the move from treatment to palliative care. Discussions become more difficult, raising challenging ethical matters.[20] In most cases, ethical treatment decisions should be shared between medical professionals and the patient.

Caring for elderly cancer patients is full of ethical issues. In fact, caring for elderly is an ethical enterprise itself, because it is value-loaded and reflects how we think about what is good in relation to health and illness, life and death. The more we are confronted with the care of elderly cancer patients, the more we will need to ask ourselves whether our current ethical approaches are sufficiently helpful in finding out what is good care in a particular situation.

FROM MEDICAL ETHICS TO ETHICS OF CARE

In this article the authors reflect on ethical issues related to cancer in the elderly. They introduce a perspective that is different from the medical ethical approach predominant in contemporary medicine, the approach of principlism. According to principlism, ethical issues are analyzed through the lens of four ethical principles that may be conflicting: respect for autonomy, beneficence, nonmaleficence, and justice.[21] The great advantage of principlism is that it provides a simple and handy tool to quickly frame ethical issues. However, there are some questions to be raised with regard to principlism. The authors name three.

First is the question of to what extent the simple framework of the four principles is equally suitable to all categories of patients. Because of its abstract nature, principlism neglects the enormous variety of patient contexts, which are often extremely meaningful to patients and hence morally relevant. Second, because of the pragmatic approach of principlism, all attention is focused on the acute problem, which is isolated from the larger context of a person's life. After the problem has been solved life continues, and many times in the case of elderly, it continues with a number of problems. One might ask whether isolating and solving separate moral problems can be considered good care. Third, principle ethics is not concerned with different versions of concepts, for example autonomy, that various participants in a moral conflict might use. Principlism's presupposition is that we all know what autonomy is, whereas it might be different for different people, as the authors illustrate.

In order to widen the moral horizon and increase moral sensitivity, in this article the authors introduce an alternative ethical framework that they consider more apt for dealing with elderly patients with cancer. This framework stems from the ethics of care, an ethical approach that focuses on the caring relationship as being constituted of both patient and professional.[22] The ethics of care approach is introduced and demonstrated by discussing two cases that are both analyzed first from the perspective of principle ethics and subsequently from the perspective of ethics of care.

Case 1: Mr Michelson

Mr Michelson is 74 years old and was admitted in the hospital for severe pneumonia. He had been ill for a long time. For 3 months he stayed in bed because he was suffering from shortness of breath. Mr Michelson is married and has three children and five grandchildren. His wife has been taking care of him and helped him with daily activities.

Mr Michelson had been diagnosed with emphysema and diabetes. He has smoked cigarettes for a long time. As concerns the cause of his pneumonia, Mr Michelson believes someone in his neighborhood infected him. The pulmonologist will do a total examination because he believes there may be something wrong. This makes Mr Michelson very upset, and he cannot sleep. After some days the diagnoses is made: non–small cell bronchus cancer and metastasis. Operation is not possible any more, but there is an option: chemotherapy. The therapy could stop growing tumor cells, and therefore offer the possibility of living a few months longer in better condition. Mr Michelson is not sure about undergoing the chemotherapy. One of his daughters insists he should take this opportunity. In the end, he decides to undergo the therapy.

While Mr Michelson undergoes the chemotherapy he has severe complications from the cytostatic. Two months after the treatment he dies. He was very weak and was admitted to the hospital. Before he died, he told the nurse that he only took the treatment for his daughter, not for himself. If he had known what chemotherapy would do to his body, he would rather have died earlier than take the treatment.

When Mr Michelson's case is analyzed from the perspective of principlism, one is inclined to focus on respect for autonomy and ask oneself how it relates to the concept of beneficence or nonmaleficence. Concerns might be raised on two levels. First, to what extent in the communication with the physician did Mr Michelson not feel pressure to undergo therapy that eventually would not be helpful to him? Looking back, one might conclude that the preconditions for informed consent were inadequately met and the physician's desire to do well so dominant that Mr Michelson's autonomy was overruled. And second, to what extent did Mr Michelson's daughter inhibit him from following his own choice?

This focus on Mr Michelson's autonomy makes sense within the framework of principlism, a course often used in ethical deliberation. Considering, however, the profile of an elderly cancer patient like Mr Michelson, who was vulnerable in physical (suffering from cancer, comorbidity, and polypharmacy), mental (cognitive decline), social (the support of his wife and children), and existential (facing death) respects, one might wonder whether it is sufficient for good care to focus on the moment of decision-making alone. Suffering is always a multidimensional process that directly affects the person as a whole.[23]

In order to get a richer view of what is ethically at stake, ethics of care might provide a useful framework of interpretation. Originally stemming from feminist discussions in the early 1980s, ethics of care posed some critical questions to contemporary culture and philosophy. Ethics of care derives its name from placing the phenomenon of care at the center of ethical reflection, noting that human existence is characterized by all kinds of informal care that is undervalued as well as important to well-being. Professional care is considered a formalized activity that is always embedded in larger social practices and relational networks. It is these latter networks that provide the particular context in which the moral good can be discovered. Thus, ethics of care places individual actions of health care professionals in a broader framework of attentiveness, responsibility, competence, and responsiveness.[24] Moreover, ethics of care is characterized by different moral presuppositions and interests, as **Table 1** demonstrates.[25]

Interpreting the case of Mr Michelson from an ethics of care perspective, one of the first questions one may ask is to what extent the choice of chemotherapy has been considered within the larger framework of his appreciation of life. Having cancer is always an existential issue. Especially when there are no options for a cure, one is confronted by one's own mortality; not in the abstract, but in a concrete and inescapable way. One of the principal characteristics of the ethics of care approach is that humans need to face their mortality and vulnerability. The idea

Table 1	
Medical ethics versus ethics of care	
Medical Ethics	**Ethics of Care**
Focus on universalizability of ethical choices and abstraction of particular patients and situations.	Focus on the uniqueness of every human being and the particularity of every situation.
Focus on freedom and autonomy: client-centeredness.	Focus on dependence and asymmetric relations of power within human relationships (professional or private).
Focus on cure: fighting disease, aging, vulnerability, suffering, and death.	Recognition and acceptance of the vulnerability of human beings.
Approach of human beings as independent individuals.	Focus on human beings as relational beings needing interpersonal relationships in order to be able to flourish.

Data from Van Heijst JE. Iemand zien staan. Zorgethiek over erkenning. Kampen (The Netherlands): Klement; 2008 [in Dutch].

that we are mortal may seem obvious. But in the reality of hospital wards, mortality is often not considered. Such an attitude is understandable from the standpoint that hospitals are focused on curing and are action-oriented. The urge to do everything that can be done is overwhelmingly strong, even if nothing at all can be done. Dealing with fatal diseases confronts both patients and caregivers with their own vulnerability and impotence. It is understandable that both caregivers and patients tend to reach to treatment in all cases in order to avoid feeling defeated or like they are giving up.[26,27]

This idea leads directly to Mr Michelson's relational network. Special attention to a patient's relational network is not exclusive to ethics of care. It is also a characteristic of a palliative care approach. Technically speaking, Mr Michelson is a palliative patient. According to the World Health Organization definition, palliative care focuses on both the patient and the family. In this case it is apparent that Mr Michelson's imminent death affects not only himself but also his wife and children. Thus it is reasonable that in this decision process, more than one voice and more than one perspective is relevant. The relational dimension of autonomy comes to the fore. The human self is inherently relational, both in the way self-consciousness develops and how it functions in later life.[28] This relationship works in two directions: from Mr Michelson to his wife and children and vice versa.

The process of saying goodbye and letting go of life is a complex one in which all close relationships enter a process of various persons following different courses and timing. Looking at the case of Mr M through the lens of care, the focus shifts from the limited role of the medical specialist in determining whether chemotherapy is in accordance with the patient's choice to the larger picture of a family confronted with the imminent death of their loved 74-year father, husband, and grandpa. Mr Michelson seems to have sensed this when he agreed to go along with his daughter's proposal. But his daughter might have been helped to distinguish between her own feelings of sadness, attachment, and impotence on the one hand and the well-being of her father on the other.

One might argue that it is not the task of a medical specialist to initiate a conversation between the patient and his or her family. From the perspective of ethics of care, however, it is precisely this broader perspective that does full justice to the process of this individual elder patient who is socially, emotionally, and existentially embedded in the context of his family. Only within this context and process can the decision to undergo another treatment or not be judged ethically good or not. Only within this context is the complex and particular situation of the elderly cancer patient dealt with in the best way.

Case 2: Mrs Johnson

Mrs Johnson is 76 years old and was diagnosed with mitral valve insufficiency 2 years ago. In the last weeks she has had difficulty walking. She could walk only small distances, and afterward she was short of breath and her heartbeat went up. She has edema of her legs. Her autonomy is going down; she is dependent on transfer, bathing, and dressing; and she is unable to do any housekeeping. She wants an operation very badly because in her opinion this is not the quality of life she wants to live with. Besides mitral insufficiency, no other comorbidities are reported.

Mrs Johnson is married and has two daughters and two grandsons. She lives with her husband in a home for the elderly and receives some housekeeping assistance once a week.

After her last visit to the cardiologist she was admitted to the hospital for a mitral valve replacement. The admission was on a Friday. All the preparations for open heart surgery had been made, and the youngest medical student was given the opportunity to examine her thoroughly for the last time. After this examination the medical student told her to stay in bed until he came back. He returned accompanied by the cardiologist, who told her that the operation would be postponed because something possibly alarming had been found in her breast. Before the heart operation could take place, the medical team wanted to know more about the finding in her breast. But because it was almost the end of the day, there was not time to do a total examination and laboratory tests. As a result, Mrs Johnson was released from the hospital until Monday.

Mrs Johnson was astonished and she objected, but she had no other option than to agree. There was not even a moment for a discussion. What could she say? The decision had been made, and she had to wait for a phone call from the hospital on Monday. Her husband and daughters wanted to tell the cardiologist what it meant for the patient and her family members to go home in this state, but they also had to wait until Monday.

On Monday Mrs Johnson received a phone call from the hospital for admission the same day, and the next day the operation would follow. The cardiologist and his team had decided that they could not postpone the operation any longer because her condition was getting worse every day, and after a short time any operation would become impossible.

Today, 10 years later, Mrs Johnson is 86 years old. Her husband died 5 years ago. She is doing well. Ten years earlier she had been the only one who knew that there was a tumour in her breast. Her mother had died of breast cancer when she was a little girl. At the time of her operation she had decided not to tell anyone because she wanted to opt for quality of life and move on. She had been afraid that if she had told the cardiologist about her lump a heart operation would not have taken place. After the heart operation she never gave permission to examine her breast. The tumour in her breast has remained the same ever since.

What is the ethical dilemma in Mrs Johnson's case? Or rather, is there a dilemma at all? Apparently from the cardiologist's perspective, there was a dilemma. Heart surgery is an invasive, high-risk intervention that is demanding for a patient in terms of energy needed for recovery. One would like to know the exact condition of the patient to be able to make a correct judgment as to whether one is not doing more damage than good. On the other hand, waiting to perform the heart surgery would put the patient in even more danger. Therefore from the perspective of principlism, the ethical demand of beneficence outweighed the demand of nonmaleficence. So far so good. Or not so good?

From an ethics of care perspective, however, the case has a different outlook. Taking the caring relationship as a social practice, it is unthinkable to postpone without discussion an operation for which a patient and her family have been preparing for weeks. Being delivered into the hands of strangers who are going to perform a high-risk invasive intervention is more than bringing one's car to the garage. It is an existential issue that touches on fundamental moral values like confidence, trust, and security, which are the basis of a happy life in general and the physician patient-relationship in particular. This patient perspective is well-adopted by caregivers who have been patients themselves. Such caregivers are very aware of the great asymmetries in the relationship between caregivers and patients.[29]

What raises ethical questions about this case is the fact that this elderly patient was prepared to be overruled by her physician. For this reason she had decided to tell no one beforehand what she had discovered in her breast. And what is worse, she was confirmed in her lack of trust and confidence by the way her operation was cancelled without discussion.

As discussed previously, an ethics of care perspective focuses on care as a process involving the caregiver's attentiveness, responsibility, competence, and responsiveness. In Mrs Johnson's case we see a lack of attentiveness and responsiveness from the side of the caregivers, however responsible and competent they believe themselves to be. In the end however, responsibility and competence without attentiveness and responsiveness can never be good care because without attentiveness and responsiveness, care does not begin and end with the patient, the vulnerable other human being who is delivered into one's professional hands.

Of course, one could object that from a caregiver's perspective the most important thing is to be sure that Mrs Johnson is being treated in a safe way. And from that perspective she could be reproached for not having told the physician about what she felt in her breast. But that reasoning is very much from the traditional caregiver's perspective. From an ethics of care perspective, care is a social practice that is constituted of both caregiver and care receiver. Ultimately it is the care receiver's vulnerable position that should guide any ethical appraisal and approach of a caring practice.

SUMMARY

In this article the authors have introduced specific characteristics of the increasingly large group of elderly cancer patients. They have argued that in order to provide good care we should extend our ethical awareness from issues of decision-making to a broader perspective focusing on the care relationship as developed by ethics of care principles. Cases like Mr. Michelson's and Mrs Johnson's show to what extent contemporary medicine is inclined to pursue its own goals of trying to do well, however taking the care receiver's perspective into account too little. An ethics of care approach may help to be more attentive and responsive to the patient's perspective. In the case of elderly cancer patients, being attentive and responsive to the patient's perspective seems to be a major precondition for delivering good quality care attuned to the need, perspective, and vulnerable position of patients.

REFERENCES

1. United Nations. World population prospects; the 2010 revision. New York; 2010.

2. Dutch Cancer Society. Cancer in the Netherlands until 2020. Amsterdam: Almedeon bv; Oisterwijk. Dutch Cancer Society; 2011.
3. Garssen J, Hoogenboezem J. Cancer mortality higher, but risk of dying from cancer lower. Statistics Netherlands; 2011.
4. Colussi AM, Mazzer L, Candotto D, et al. The elderly cancer patient: a nursing perspective. Crit Rev Oncol Hematol 2001;39:235–45.
5. Janssen J. Communicating with older cancer patients: impact on information recall. Netherlands Institute for Health Services Research: Utrecht (The Netherlands); 2009.
6. Overcash J, Balduci L. The older cancer patient. A guide for nurses and related professionals. New York: Springer Publishing Company Inc; 2003.
7. de Vries M, van Weert JC, Jansen J, et al. Step by step development of clinical care pathways for older cancer patients: necessary or desirable? Eur J Cancer 2007;43: 2170–8.
8. Maas H. Unravelling heterogeneity in elder cancer patients. Rotterdam (The Netherlands): Erasmus University; 2011.
9. De Rijke JM. Cancer in the elderly. Maastricht (The Netherlands): Maastricht University; 2003.
10. Extermann M. Interaction between comorbidity and cancer. Cancer Control 2007;14: 13–22.
11. Holmes HM. Staging the Aging: geriatricians help older patients choose cancer treatment. Spring: University of Texas Anderson Network; 2011.
12. Repetto L, Venturino A, Fratino L, et al. Geriatric oncology: a clinical approach to the older patient with cancer. Eur J Cancer 2003;39:870–80.
13. Silvestri G, Pritchard RS, Welch HG. Preferences for chemotherapy in patients with advanced non-small cell lung cancer; descriptive study based on descriptive interventions. BMJ 1998;317(7161):1771–5.
14. Bremnes RM, Andersen K, Wist EA. Cancer patients doctors and nurses vary in their willingness to undertake cancer chemotherapy. Eur J Cancer 1995;31A(12):1955–9.
15. Extermann M, Hurria A. Comprehensive geriatric assessment for older patients with cancer. J Clin Oncol 2007;25:1824–31.
16. Maas HA, Janssen-Heijnen ML, Olde Rikkert MG, et al. Comprehensive geriatric assessment and its clinical impact in oncology. Eur J Cancer 2007;43:261–9.
17. Klepin H, Mohile SG, Hurria A. Geriatric assessment in older patients with breast cancer. J Natl Compr Canc Netw 2009;7:226–36.
18. Gobbens R. Frail elderly. Towards an integral approach. Tilburg (The Netherlands): Tilburg University; 2010.
19. Gobbens R. Frail elderly. Towards an integral approach. Verpleegkunde Nederlands Vlaams Wetenschappelijk Tijdschrift 2010;3:25.
20. Gallanger A, Gannon C. Difficult decisions in cancer care - conducting an ethic case analyses. European Oncology & Haematology, 2011;7(2):101–5.
21. Beauchamp T, Childress J. Principles of biomedical ethics. New York: Oxford University Press; 2001.
22. Held V. The ethics of care. In: Copp D, editor. Oxford handbook of ethical theory. New York: Oxford University Press; 2006. p. 537–66.
23. Cassell E. The nature of suffering and the goals of medicine. 2nd edition. New York: Oxford University Press; 2004.
24. Tronto JC. Moral boundaries. A political argument for an ethic of care. New York: Routledge; 1993.
25. Van Heijst JE. Iemand zien staan. Zorgethiek over erkenning. Kampen (The Netherlands): Klement; 2008 [in Dutch].

26. Van Laarhoven H, Leget C, Van der Graaf W. Dying at the right time: a modern dilemma. Oncologist 2009;14:642–3.
27. Van Laarhoven H, Leget C, Van der Graaf W. When hope is all there is left. Oncologist 2011;16:914–6.
28. Ricoeur P. Oneself as another. Chicago: University of Chicago Press; 1992.
29. Klitzman R. When doctors become patients. New York: Oxford University Press; 2008.

The Use of Radiation Therapy in the Geriatric Population

Benjamin Rosenbluth, MD

KEYWORDS
- Geriatric • Cancer • Treatment • Radiation therapy

As the medical community has developed increasingly effectual treatments for illnesses and conditions that once claimed the lives of younger patients, including heart disease, diabetes, and infectious diseases, we have seen the average life expectancy in the United States rise significantly. Such welcome news is accompanied, however, by an increase in the incidence of diseases more prevalent in the elderly population, including cancer. We are therefore faced more frequently with the clinical problem of how best to approach the care of the elderly cancer patient.

BASICS OF RADIATION DELVERY

Radiation therapy (RT) is often used as a fundamental component of the treatment of patients with cancer. It may be used in conjunction with chemotherapy or surgery, but it may also be used on its own, in clinically appropriate scenarios, for either palliative or curative purposes.

RT consists of the focusing of high-energy particles, often photons or electrons, on a specific part of the anatomy. The high-energy particles are believed to cause preferential tumor-cell death primarily via DNA damage; tumor cells are less able to repair than normal-tissue cells. However, RT is certainly able to cause damage to normal tissue cells as well, especially if given in sufficiently high doses. Therefore, to maximize the therapeutic window, RT is typically "fractionated," or given as multiple smaller doses, usually delivered daily (Monday through Friday). This smaller daily dose enables normal healthy tissues to repair themselves, an activity in which tumor cells are relatively deficient.

In general, treatment with radiation is painless and is similar to undergoing a diagnostic x-ray. However, to ensure accurate treatment delivery, very precise immobilization and positioning techniques are generally used. Thus, more time is

The author has nothing to disclose.
Department of Radiation Oncology, Holy Name Medical Center, 718 Teaneck Road, Teaneck, NJ 07666, USA
E-mail address: bdrosenbluth@yahoo.com

Clin Geriatr Med 28 (2012) 105–114
doi:10.1016/j.cger.2011.12.001
0749-0690/12/$ – see front matter © 2012 Elsevier Inc. All rights reserved.

often spent "setting up" the patient in the appropriate treatment position than in actually delivering the treatment, which may only take a few minutes.

GENERAL CONSIDERATIONS REGARDING THE USE OF RADIATION THERAPY IN THE ELDERLY

Elderly oncology patients are often not offered therapy due to concerns about their age.[1,2] However, multiple studies have shown that age ought not be the deciding factor in determining whether RT should be offered.[3] In fact, RT may be particularly useful in the treatment of elderly patients when surgery and chemotherapy are contraindicated, given the noninvasive and anatomically localized nature of RT.

Instead of chronologic age, it has been more effective to consider patients' physiologic age when considering them for RT, as well as chemotherapy or surgery. A very young patient with multiple comorbidities as at far greater risk of complication due to cancer treatment than is an older patient with good activity and energy levels. At our center, we use the Karnofsky Performance Scale (KPS) in all oncologic patient assessments, and this frequently helps determine how aggressively cancer treatment should be pursued.

Another tool that has been found to be helpful for determining elderly patients' functional status has been the Comprehensive Geriatric Assessment (CGA). In addition to the patient's functional status, the CGA estimates the presence of comorbidities, mental status, emotional conditions, social support, nutritional status, polypharmacy, and the presence of geriatric syndromes.[4,5]

A major advantage of RT over systemic therapy is the locoregional nature of the treatment. With proper planning and delivery, RT can treat very specific areas and essentially avoid any damage to organs outside the irradiated field. In addition, with attentive and aggressive management, even locoregional side effects can be effectively treated and often prevented altogether. Thus, RT can be beneficial to elderly patients even when systemic therapy or surgery is contraindicated. However, concurrent chemoradiation must often be approached with extreme caution in these patients, and dose reduction of chemotherapy must be used at times to reduce toxic side effects.[6]

POTENTIAL DIFFICULTIES IN TREATMENT OF THE GERIATRIC POPULATION WITH RADIATION THERAPY

It should be pointed out, however, that consideration of potential toxicities in certain organs, even in the absence of concurrent chemotherapy, may play a role in the management and possibly the use of RT in elderly patients. RT to the whole brain, often performed for palliative or prophylactic purposes, may produce long-term neurocognitive deficits.[7] Thus, the neurocognitive function of an elderly patient with baseline symptoms of dementia may be further exacerbated with whole brain RT, and the potential benefits of such therapy must be carefully weighed against the potential problems it may cause. In addition, pelvic RT may cause bone marrow suppression and gastrointestinal or urinary side effects, which may necessitate careful monitoring and response in patients who are, for example, cytopenic or prone to anorexia, dehydration, or urinary difficulties.

One of the most common challenges in the use of RT for the elderly is the length of the course of treatment. Traditionally, a course of definitive RT might last anywhere from 5 to 9 weeks. For patients who are not able to drive, this can be daunting, and without family, friends, or hired hands to bring the patient to the clinic, it is essentially impossible to commit to a full course of treatment. Although it is potentially more realistic to plan on completing a palliative course of RT, which may lasts a shorter 1 to 3 weeks, immobile patients are challenged by such a situation as well.

The length of individual treatments may pose challenges, albeit minor ones, for elderly patients. It may occasionally be difficult for patients to maintain the same position for treatment for an extended length of time. Patients with congestive heart failure, for example, especially those who are oxygen dependent, may have a difficult time lying supine, which is the position in which patients are treated most frequently. These patients often require particularly expeditious care, with minimization of their time spent in the treatment position.

Patients may need to raise their arms to prevent interference with the radiation beam, and this position, especially for extended lengths of time, may become uncomfortable. In truth, these concerns appear to occur with the same frequency in the younger and older populations, although one might anticipate otherwise. We have found prophylactic treatment with nonsteroidal anti-inflammatory drugs to be particularly useful for these patients.

Ironically, for particularly disabled patients, such as those whose condition has forced them to live in assisted living facilities, transportation is often less of a challenge, as ambulances regularly work with such facilities to bring the patients to and from the RT center daily.

RECENT ADVANCES IN RADIATION THERAPY PLANNING AND DELIVERY

Fortunately, recent advances in treatment precision, accuracy, and technology have enabled many treatments, both definitive and palliative, to be delivered over significantly shorter periods of time, and often with less discomfort to the patient. Early stage lung cancer, for example, has shown phenomenal responsiveness to treatment using stereotactic body radiosurgery (SBRT), in which a full course of definitive therapy, with outcomes rivaling even those of conventional surgery, can be delivered within 1 to 2 weeks' time.

In fact, when used in other organs, SBRT techniques have enabled an entire treatment course to be delivered in as little as a single treatment. This has been particularly useful for palliative treatment, such as for bone metastases. However, even when performed over 3 to 5 fractions, SBRT results have been impressive, in terms of both local control as well as toxicity, and require fewer visits to a treatment center. In addition to the treatment of both primary and oligometastatic lung tumors, SBRT has been shown to play a potential role in the treatment of gynecologic malignancies.[8] Higginson and colleagues reviewed their own experience, in addition to those of other institutions, with using SBRT for gynecologic malignancies. They treated 16 gynecologic patients with SBRT, including to the pelvic and periaortic nodes (9 patients), to oligometastatic disease (2), and to cervical or endometrial primary tumors when other conventional external radiation or brachytherapy techniques were unsuitable (5). Median preliminary follow-up was 11 months, and they found 79% locoregional control, 43% distant failure, and 50% overall survival rates. The use of SBRT helped attenuate traditional concerns related to the proximity of periaortic nodes to small bowel, which often precluded the use of more conventional RT. Data such as these suggest increasing applicability of SBRT for multiple disease site, with better outcomes and shorter treatment times. Thus, older patients, who may be an unacceptable surgical risk, even for a minor procedure such as a brachytherapy application, would still be candidates for higher conformal and potentially curative radiosurgical approaches.

It should be noted, however, that SBRT does require very precise immobilization and the use of multiple noncoplanar radiation beams, which may add somewhat to the time spent on the treatment table per fraction. In our experience, however, patient dissatisfaction related to time spent on the treatment table for an SBRT treatment was not directly related to patient age but rather to patient comorbidities (eg, arthritis). This again argues in favor of using the CGA, along with other performance status assessments, in the evaluation of a patient's appropriateness for various treatments.

Fortunately, recent technological advances, including Varian's RapidArc technology (Varian Medical Systems, Inc., Palo Alto, CA, USA), have been shown to enable complex organ-sparing treatment plans such as SBRT to be delivered in a significantly shorter time period, thus decreasing the patient's time spent in the treatment position. This may very well further broaden the number of patients who can tolerate a course of SBRT. In addition, recent reports, such as that from Kuo and colleagues,[9] have demonstrated favorable tumor coverage using RapidArc plan for primary hepatocellular carcinoma compared with 3-dimensional conformal radiotherapy and intensity-modulated radiotherapy (IMRT) plans. Studies have also shown RapidArc to be equivalent or superior to IMRT for other malignancies, including head and neck cancer and prostate cancer.[10–12] Thus, RapidArc is becoming recognized as a potentially more efficient and more effective treatment option for patients and would hopefully provide greater opportunity particularly for elderly patients to receive a full course of treatment.

SITE-SPECIFIC CONSIDERATIONS

Certain disease sites require specific age-related considerations, regarding tumor aggressiveness, treatment efficacy, and treatment-related toxicity. Breast cancer, for example, has shown a general decrease in aggressive behavior with increasing age of the patient at the time of diagnosis. Women over 70 years of age with early-stage hormone-sensitive breast tumors, in particular, have been shown to have a significantly decreased rate of local recurrence, compared to younger patients, even without the use of adjuvant RT, although postoperative RT does still decrease the rate of local recurrence, from approximately 4% to 1%, when given in conjunction with surgery and tamoxifen.[13]

In addition, for such patients, a more convenient form of adjuvant RT, known as accelerated partial breast irradiation (APBI), has been found to be quite effective and involves only 1 week of treatment. This treatment is usually delivered twice a day for 5 consecutive days and may be delivered using either conformal external radiation techniques or a high-dose–rate catheter-based afterloading system, which requires perioperative placement by the surgeon of a percutaneous catheter in the region of the tumor bed. APBI has been a particularly attractive option for elderly patients, for whom transportation is often more of a problem.[14]

Another recent technique for adjuvant breast cancer RT involves the use of traditional external beam techniques to deliver a somewhat higher dose per day so that the overall number of treatment days may be decreased, while maintaining an appropriate biologically effective dose. One of the more widely accepted dose-fractionation schemes to accomplish this, developed and validated by Whelan and colleagues, decreases the overall treatment time from approximately 5 weeks to approximately 3 weeks. This technique has been dubbed "Canadian fractionation," in reference to Dr Whelan's geographic location.[15]

There has been some reversal in the approach to the use of the traditional "boost" portion of a typical course of postoperative breast radiation as part of a breast-conserving therapy approach. For most patients, following an approximately 5-week course of whole-breast RT, a shorter, approximately 1-week "boost" course of RT is delivered to the lumpectomy cavity plus a small margin. This is to address the elevated likelihood of local recurrence in the region of the initial lumpectomy. A boost-versus-no-boost trial was performed by the EORTC[15] and revealed that the 5-year local-control benefit of the boost, while apparent in all age groups, was less significant in the older ago groups. Thus, in patients over the age of 60, the breast boost was often omitted.

This decision had the added benefit of shortening the length of the overall RT course for these elderly patients. However, when these data were updated with 10-year follow-up, the magnitude of the relative risk reduction due to the boost was found to be significant in all age groups, though the absolute risk reduction of local recurrence remained greatest in the younger age group.[16]

Uterine cancer, unlike breast cancer, potentially exhibits more aggressive behavior in the older population. Recent SEER (Surveillance, Epidemiology and End Results) data have suggested that there is increased survival seen in younger endometrial cancer patients.[17] The NCCN (National Comprehensive Cancer Network) guidelines for the treatment of endometrial cancer have, in fact, incorporated age as one of the "potential adverse risk factors" influencing, in turn, the advisability of observation versus vaginal brachytherapy versus external beam pelvic RT as adjuvant treatment following the diagnosis of completely surgically staged stage I disease.[18]

There have been other tumor sites in which advanced age has been shown to act as a negative prognostic factor. In the case of high-grade glioma, for instance, patients older than 65 years have shown consistently worse outcomes.[19]

RECENT EFFORTS AT EVALUATING USE OF RADIATION THERAPY IN THE ELDERLY

With increased interest in the management of cancer in the geriatric population, there have been several recent studies evaluating patterns of use of various treatment modalities in elderly oncologic patients. Horiot performed an excellent review of multiple studies, all of which had been designed, at least in part, to aid in understanding the geriatric population's tolerance of RT.[20]

Horiot reported the results of Bouvier and colleagues,[21] who studied the outcomes of 838 rectal cancers treated in patients 80 years and older. He estimated that at least 50% of the clinical situations justified RT in a similar group of younger age patients but noted that, in fact, only 17% of the elderly group received RT. He noted that 73% of the patients underwent surgery, suggesting good general condition, and confirming significant underuse of RT in this elderly population.

More recently, Quipourt and colleagues[22] evaluated 2921 colorectal cancers diagnosed between 2004 and 2007 and noted that RT was administered in 59.0% of patients aged 75 and older with rectal cancer, versus 85.3% of those younger than 75 ($P<.01$). Thus, while the use of RT has mostly increased, likely as a result of the randomized Swedish trials showing a survival benefit for preoperative RT in moderately advanced rectal cancer patients, the difference in use of RT between older and younger patients has remained.

In his review, Horiot also reported on 3 reviews of the relationship between age at presentation and clinical outcomes of patients treated within EORTC (European Organization for Research and Treatment of Cancer) RT protocols. These protocols were performed in 1996, 1997, and 1998 and included 4406 patients with head and neck, pelvic, and thoracic cancers.[23–25] He noted no impact of age in outcomes after radical RT for head and neck tumors, aside from more severe functional acute reactions in the older patients. There was also no difference seen in survival between age groups treated for prostate, uterus, and anal cancer. Rectal cancer alone was associated with a significantly improved survival in younger patients. Thus, the conclusion was that, with the exception of rectal cancer, age is not a limiting factor for radical RT in pelvic malignancies. Among bronchial cancer, there was only found to be a trend toward increased weight loss in older patients following radical RT. Thus, the recommendation was made that future RT protocols for these anatomic sites not include an upper age limit.

Horiot reviewed 31 EORTC RT protocols that had been recruiting since 1995 and found that, while the inclusion of the age group 65 to 70 years was well accepted, extension of entry beyond age 70 remained unsuccessful in most tumor sites. Overall, more than half (57%) of the protocols activated after 1995 had followed the EORTC recommendation to delete age limits in RT protocols.

A review of currently open RTOG (Radiation Therapy Oncology Group) trials reveals no upper age limits in the eligibility criteria for enrollment.

MORE RECENT SITE-SPECIFIC STUDIES

In recent years, a number of investigators have reported on the response of elderly patients to RT for treatment of various sites. Pallis and colleagues[26] reported on the use of combined chemoradiotherapy for elderly patients with small cell lung cancer in multiple trials. When standard combined chemoradiotherapy approaches for limited-stage disease were evaluated, the toxicity and overall survival data were conflicting, and a tendency toward less aggressive use of chemotherapy or RT in the elderly was noted. The authors concluded that while standard approaches are feasible in carefully selected elderly patients, more data from elderly-specific clinical trials will be necessary to provide evidence-based recommendations for the treatment of the geriatric population. They did note as well that data suggest CGA procedures should be used more frequently in everyday clinical practice.

Tougeron and colleagues[27] evaluated the tolerance and outcome of patients older than 70 years treated with chemoradiotherapy for esophageal cancer. One hundred nine patients were investigated and a 57.8% clinical complete response rate and 35.5% 2-year survival rate were observed, while adverse events grade 3 or worse were seen in 23.8% of patients. These results suggested a similar response rate and overall survival compared to those seen in younger patients treated with the same regimen. Local recurrence and metastasis rates were also in accordance with prior randomized trials. The authors conclude that definitive chemoradiotherapy could be considered as an effective treatment with no significant toxicity in elderly patients with esophageal cancer.

Tougeron and colleagues[28] have also reviewed the outcomes of 125 patients with rectal cancer between 70 and 90 years old who were treated with chemoradiotherapy in 2 French university hospitals. Adverse effects of grade 2 or greater were observed in 32% of patients and adverse effects of grade 3 or greater in 15%. Dose reduction due to toxicity occurred in 18% of the patients and chemoradiotherapy was discontinued in 9%. Postoperative morbidity was 16% with 2 treatment-related deaths. Two-year survival rate was 84%. The authors concluded that, in selected elderly patients, chemoradiotherapy is well tolerated, without significant increase in adverse events. They also noted that results are similar to those recorded in younger patients.

Hsieh and colelagues[29] reported on their results using post-TURBT (transurethral resection of bladder tumor) intensity-modulated radiation therapy (IMRT) and helical tomotherapy (HT) for elderly patients with bladder cancer. The median age was 80 (range, 65 to 90) years. They reported a median survival of 21 months. The 2-year overall survival was 26.3% (IMRT group) and 37.5% (HT group), disease-free survival was 58.3% (IMRT group) and 83.3% (HT group), locoregional progression-free survival was 87.5% (IMRT group) and 83.3% (HT group), and metastasis-free survival was 66.7% (IMRT group) and 35.4% (HT group). They also noted a significantly worse 2-year overall survival rate for patients whose RT completion time was greater than 8 weeks compared to those who completed RT within 8 weeks (37.9% vs 0%). They concluded that IMRT and HT provide good locoregional progression-free survival with tolerable toxicity for elderly patients with invasive bladder cancer.

Jensen and colleagues[30] described their experience treating 73 patients with primary or recurrent squamous cell carcinoma of the head and neck (SCCHN) with RT and cetuximab. The overall response rate was 59.4%, the median locoregional and overall progression-free survival rates were 18 and 15 months, and the overall survival rate was 18 months. They concluded that this treatment regimen is a feasible treatment option for elderly and multimorbid patients with promising therapeutic activity.

When treating 380 patients with squamous cell carcinoma of the uterine cervix with a combination of external beam therapy and 3 brachytherapy fractions, Sakurai and colleagues[31] found no statistical significance in the 5-year intrapelvic recurrence rates among patients under 70 years old, 70 to 79 years old, and 80 years or older. This course of definitive treatment was concluded to be both highly effective and safe for senior patients with cervical squamous cell carcinoma.

Hayakawa and colleagues[32] retrospectively analyzed 97 patients aged 75 years or older with inoperable or unresectable non–small cell lung cancer (NSCLC) and compared them with 206 patients younger than 75 years. Most patients were treated with a total dose of 60 Gy or more in 2-Gy daily standard fractionation. No statistically significant difference in survival rates was seen, although the post-treatment deterioration rate of performance status was only 5% in the younger group and 8% in the elderly group. Only 3 younger and 2 elderly patients died of late pulmonary insufficiency associated with high-dose irradiation to the proximal bronchus. No other treatment-related event was observed except for mild acute complications in the elderly groups. The authors thus recommended that definitive RT be offered to the elderly aged 75 years or older with inoperable or unresectable NSCLC as an acceptable choice of treatment.

OTHER OBSERVATIONAL STUDIES OF INTEREST

Nikolaou and Pangali[33] performed an interesting prospective, descriptive study investigating differences between younger (less than 65 years) and older (65 years or older) RT patients with regard to the rates of comorbidities, polypharmacy, and the cost of drug prescription. Two hundred outpatients were enrolled. Not unexpectedly, older patients had a higher rate of comorbidity and had been prescribed more medications for the management of comorbid disorders. However, during RT, the younger group was found to need more "supportive care medications" (ie, medications prescribed as a result of complications or toxicity encountered during RT). This resulted in a higher mean total medication cost per patient in the younger group. Interestingly, the reported toxicity rates and severity for the 2 groups during RT were similar. This finding was perhaps related to a previously reported finding that younger patients report more concerns about their illness and symptoms.[34]

Mitsuhashi and colleagues[35] reported on the clinical efficacy of RT in general for patients aged 90 years or older. They retrospectively analyzed 32 patients (11 men, 21 women) aged 90 years or older who underwent radiation therapy in 1970–1997. Head and neck cancer (n = 14 [44%]) and skin cancer (n = 6 [19%]) were the most common cancers treated in this group. Eleven (79%) of the 14 patients with head and neck cancer were treated with curative intent. Radiation response without any severe complication was observed in 9 (90%) of the 10 patients with head and neck cancer treated with curative intent who finished treatment. The median survival time was 8 months in these 10 patients. Complete response was achieved in all patients with skin cancer without any major sequelae. Complete response was also observed in all 3 the patients with non-Hodgkin lymphoma, but 2 patients treated with adjuvant chemotherapy died of drug-induced pneumonitis. Palliation was achieved in all 9 patients treated with palliative intent. The authors' conclusion was that age of 90 years or older is not a limiting factor for RT. It bears mentioning that, given the years during which these patients were treated, most of these patients could not have been treated with anything approaching the modern conformal and precise techniques we have mentioned earlier. Thus, these findings are particularly hopeful regarding the future use of RT and the likely therapeutic ratio one would expect to see, even in this particularly elderly subset.

SUMMARY

The foregoing, it is hoped, has provided at least a taste of the past, present, and future in the use of RT for the elderly population. Based on many ongoing studies, it becomes clear that the radiation oncology world has come to recognize the geriatric population's ability to tolerate, and perhaps even thrive from, a course of RT, when it is offered appropriately. In the final analysis, it has become clear that no simple age cutoff can substitute for clinical acumen and a thorough assessment of patients' general health before the best treatment regimen can be chosen.

One need only follow the trend both in American and in European trials (the RTOG and the EORTC) to appreciate the acceptance that has taken hold that there need not be an age cutoff so much as a set of clinical criteria, including performance status and other assessments of function and comorbidity, prior to patient enrollment in a national trial. With such an outlook, we eagerly anticipate the results from these trials and look forward to implementing them in our treatment of young and old patients alike.

REFERENCES

1. Muss H, Longo D. Introduction: Cancer in the elderly. Semin Oncol 2004;31:125–7.
2. Fentiman I, Tirelli U, Monfardini S. Cancer in the elderly: why so badly treated? Lancet 1990;335:1020–2.
3. Zachariah B, Balducci L, Venkattarmanabalaji G. Radiotherapy for cancer patients aged 80 and older: a study of effectiveness and side effects. Int J Radiat Oncol Biol Physics 1997;39:1125.
4. Extermann M, Hurria A. Comprehensive geriatric assessment for older patients with cancer. J Clin Oncol 2007;10:1824–31.
5. Carreca I, Balducci L, Extermann M. Cancer in the older person. Cancer Treat Rev 2005;31:380–402.
6. National Comprehensive Cancer Network. NCCN Guidelines. Available at: http://www.nccn.org/professionals/physician_gls/pdf/senior.pdf. Accessed December 6, 2011.
7. Bovi JA, White J. Radiation therapy in the prevention of brain metastases. Curr Oncol Rep 2011. [Epub ahead of print].
8. Higginson DS, Morris DE, Jones EL, et al. Stereotactic body radiotherapy (SBRT): technological innovation and application in gynecologic oncology. Gynecol Oncol 2011;120:404–12.
9. Kuo YC, Chiu YM, Shih WP, et al. Volumetric intensity-modulated Arc (RapidArc) therapy for primary hepatocellular carcinoma: comparison with intensity-modulated radiotherapy and 3-D conformal radiotherapy. Radiat Oncol 2011;6:76.

10. Verbakel WF, Cuijpers JP, Hoffmans D, et al. Volumetric intensity-modulated arc therapy vs. conventional IMRT in head-and-neck cancer: a comparative planning and dosimetric study. Int J Radiat Oncol Biol Phys 2009;74:252–9.

11. Yoo S, Wu QJ, Lee WR, et al. Radiotherapy treatment plans with RapidArc for prostate cancer involving seminal vesicles and lymph nodes. Int J Radiat Oncol Biol Phys 2010;76:935–42.

12. Palma D, Vollans E, James K, et al. Volumetric modulated arc therapy for delivery of prostate radiotherapy: comparison with intensity-modulated radiotherapy and three-dimensional conformal radiotherapy. Int J Radiat Oncol Biol Phys 2008;15:72:996–1001.

13. Hughes KS, Schnaper LA, Berry D, et al. Lumpectomy plus tamoxifen with or without irradiation in women 70 years of age or older with early breast cancer. N Engl J Med. 2004;351:971–7.

14. Khan AJ, Arthur D, Vicini F, et al. Six-year analysis of treatment-related toxicities in patients treated with accelerated partial breast irradiation on the American Society of Breast Surgeons MammoSite Breast Brachytherapy Registry Trial. Ann Surg Oncol 2011. [Epub ahead of print].

15. Whelan TJ, Pignol JP, Levine MN, et al. Long-term results of hypofractionated radiation therapy for breast cancer. N Engl J Med 2010;362:513–20.

16. Poortmans PM, Collette L, Bartelink H, et al. The addition of a boost dose on the primary tumour bed after lumpectomy in breast conserving treatment for breast cancer. A summary of the results of EORTC 22881-10882 "boost versus no boost" trial. Cancer Radiother 2008;12:565–70.

17. Chan JK, Sherman AE, Kapp DS, et al. Influence of gynecologic oncologists on the survival of patients with endometrial cancer. J Clin Oncol 2011;29:832–8.

18. National Comprehensive Cancer Network. NCCN Guidelines. Available at: http://www.nccn.org/professionals/physician_gls/pdf/uterine.pdf. Accessed December 6, 2011.

19. Peschel RE, Wilson L, Haffty B, et al. The effect of advanced age on the efficacy of radiation therapy for early breast cancer, local prostate cancer and grade III–IV gliomas. Int J Radiat Oncol Biol Phys 1993;26:539–44.

20. Horiot JC. Radiation therapy and the geriatric oncology patient. J Clin Oncol 2007; 25(14):1930–5.

21. Bouvier AM, Launoy G, Lepage C, et al. Trends in the management and survival of digestive tract cancers among patients aged over 80 years. Aliment Pharmacol Ther 2005;22:233–41.

22. Quipourt V, Jooste V, Cottet V, et al. Comorbidities alone do not explain the undertreatment of colorectal cancer in older adults: a French population-based study. J Am Geriatr Soc 2011;59:694–8.

23. Pignon T, Horiot JC, Van den Bogaert W, et al. No age limit for radical radiotherapy in head and neck tumours. Eur J Cancer 1996;32A:2075–81.

24. Pignon T, Horiot JC, Bolla M, et al. Age is not a limiting factor for radical radiotherapy in pelvic malignancies. Radiother Oncol 1997;42:107–20.

25. Pignon T, Gregor A, Schaake Koning C, et al. Age has no impact on acute and late toxicity of curative thoracic radiotherapy. Radiother Oncol 1998;46:239–48.

26. Pallis AG, Shepherd FA, Lacombe D, et al. Treatment of small-cell lung cancer in elderly patients. Cancer 2010;116:1192–200.

27. Tougeron D, Di Fiore F, Thureau S, et al. Safety and outcome of definitive chemoradio-therapy in elderly patients with oesophageal cancer. Br J Cancer 2008;99:1586–92.

28. Tougeron D, Roullet B, Paillot B, et al. Safety and outcome of chemoradiotherapy in elderly patients with rectal cancer: results from two French tertiary centres. Dig Liver Dis 2011. [Epub ahead of print].

29. Hsieh CH, Chung SD, Chan PH, et al. Intensity modulated radiotherapy for elderly bladder cancer patients. Radiat Oncol 2011;6:75.

30. Jensen AD, Bergmann ZP, Garcia-Huttenlocher H, et al. Cetuximab and radiation for primary and recurrent squamous cell carcinoma of the head and neck (SCCHN) in the elderly and multi-morbid patient: a single-centre experience. Head Neck Oncol 2010;26:34.

31. Sakurai H, Mitsuhashi N, Takahashi M, et al. Radiation therapy for elderly patient with squamous cell carcinoma of the uterine cervix. Gynecol Oncol 2000;77:116–20.

32. Hayakawa K, Mitsuhashi N, Katano S, et al. High-dose radiation therapy for elderly patients with inoperable or unresectable non-small cell lung cancer. Lung Cancer 2001;32:81–8.

33. Nikolaou C, Vassiliou V, Pangali M, et al. Cost of medication requirement during radiotherapy: implications for an elderly oncological population. J Am Geriatr Soc 2007;55:958–9.

34. Turner NJ, Muers MF, Haward RA, et al. Psychological distress and concerns of elderly patients treated with palliative radiotherapy for lung cancer. Psychooncology 2007;16:707–13.

35. Mitsuhashi N, Hayakawa K, Yamakawa M, et al. Cancer in patients aged 90 years or older: radiation therapy. Radiology 1999;211:829–33.

Liquid Tumors in the Elderly

Anthony Mato, MD*, Tatyana Feldman, MD, Joshua Richter, MD, David S. Siegel, MD, PhD, Andre Goy, MD, MS

KEYWORDS

- Acute myelogenous leukemia • Acute Lymphoblastic Leukemia
- Diffuse large B-cell lymphoma • Multiple myeloma

ACUTE LEUKEMIA MANAGEMENT IN GERIATRIC MEDICINE
Acute Myelogenous Leukemia

Acute myelogenous leukemia (AML) is the most common type of acute leukemia in the United States. With a median age at diagnosis of 67 years (SEER database), AML is by definition a disease of the elderly, with the majority of cases being diagnosed in the sixth and seventh decades of life. Multiple studies suggest that increasing age is a predictor of inferior outcomes in AML. Specifically, elderly patients with AML appear to have inferior rates of complete remission (CR), duration of response, treatment-related mortality and, most importantly, overall survival.[1,2] There is no single specific cause of inferior outcomes in elderly AML, but rather, like most oncologic diseases, the etiology of poor outcomes is multifactorial, including clinical, psychological, metabolic, genetic, and biological factors, all of which can contribute to the failure of traditional treatment approaches successfully used in younger patients (age <60 years).[3]

Prognosis

Clinical risk factors, such as concurrent comorbid conditions, poor performance status, cognitive decline, lack of an available caretaker, and inadequate transportation, undoubtedly contribute to inferior results.[3] Additionally, a false perception by the medical community that all elderly patients with AML are unlikely to benefit from traditional remission induction therapy followed by postremission consolidation can lead to delays in therapy initiation or inappropriate treatment selection (dose reductions, substitutions), also contributing to failure.[3,4] Although clinical risk factors remain important contributors to poor outcomes, the data strongly suggest that inferior outcomes are in large part caused by a distinct biological profile with a

The authors have nothing to disclose.

John Theurer Cancer Center, Hackensack University Medical Center, 92 Second Street, Hackensack, NJ 07601, USA

* Corresponding author.

E-mail address: AMato@humed.com

disproportionate incidence of poor-risk, leukemia-related, prognostic factors in the geriatric population.

Using classical karyotyping methods on AML blast cells, one can risk stratify patients into distinct risk groups. Predictive cytogenetic models for risk stratification proposed by cooperative groups (Eastern Cooperative Oncology Group [ECOG]-South Western Oncology Group [SWOG], CALGB, and the Medical Research Council [MRC]) are widely used in clinical practice to stratify AML patients into so-called good risk, intermediate-risk, and poor-risk groups (ie, chromosome 5 or 7 or complex karyotypes with 3 or more abnormalities).[5–7] Poor-risk karyotypes translate clinically into inferior rates of remission, shorter duration of response, and inferior survival—independent of patient age.[5] A major limitation of this approach is that traditional cytogenetics can take several days to perform and report and, thus, may not be available at the crucial moment that a treatment decision is mandated. Unfortunately, elderly patients with AML have a disproportionate shift from favorable and intermediate cytogenetic profiles to unfavorable cytogenetic profiles (in excess of 50%), explaining in large part the inferior outcomes reported in numerous trials.[8,9] More recently, approaches using fluorescent in-situ hybridization (FISH), PCR-based assays, micro-RNA expression, flow cytometry, and gene expression profiling are being used to risk stratify patients as well as to identify new pathways to target in drug design.[10–14] These approaches (with the potential for a relatively faster turnaround time) may be particularly useful in the risk stratification of AML patients who have normal karyotypes (intermediate risk) or those without an available karyotype (ie, test not sent, cells did not grow).

Although morphologically the AML blast is not particularly distinct in elderly patients, at the level of cell biology one can detect distinct differences. One important example is an increased expression of the multidrug resistance 1 (MDR1) gene, leading to upregulation of permeability glycoprotein at the cell surface, allowing for highly efficient efflux of chemotherapy out from the AML blast leading to resistance to chemotherapy.[8–15] The presence of MDR1 upregulation is associated with lower remission rates. Several attempts have been made to overcome MDR1 resistance by increasing chemotherapy doses or combining chemotherapy with specific MDR1 inhibitors, unfortunately without demonstrating a clear clinical benefit.[16,17]

Therapy

The traditional treatment approach for remission induction (termed *3 + 7*) for patients with newly diagnosed AML includes 1 to 2 courses of combination chemotherapy of an anthracycline (usually given over 3 days) with cytarabine (usually given by continuous infusion over 7 days). Patients who are able to achieve a CR (defined as the absence of leukemic blasts seen in bone marrow or peripheral blood with concomitant normalization of hematologic indices) are candidates for consolidation therapy (potentially curative), including additional courses of chemotherapy (typically high-dose cytarabine, (HiDAC) or combination anthracycline-cytarabine) or allogeneic stem cell transplantation.[18–20]

For elderly patients, results of clinical trials have been disappointing using standard remission induction strategies.[21–23] Recent attempts to overcome the poor prognostic features of elderly AML using standard approaches have focused on dose modification. Lowenberg and colleagues[24] recently reported outcomes of 813 (age >60) AML patients treated with daunarobicin (45 mg/m^2 vs 90 mg/m^2) and cytarabine. Although increasing anthracycline dose resulted in a higher percentage of patients achieving CR (54% vs 64%) without an impact on treatment-related mortality (11% vs12%), long-term outcomes remained poor regardless of anthracycline dose with

17% versus 19% of patients alive at 5 years. Data reported by Burnett and coworkers[25] in elderly patients (1273 patients, age > 60) with newly diagnosed AML treated with daunorubicin (35 vs 50 mg/m^2) and escalated-dose cytarabine (200 vs 400 mg/m^2) did not show an increased CR rate when cytarabine dose was escalated or daunorubicin dose was reduced and highlight a 16% to 18% risk of death during induction and 11% to 13% 5-year survival rate. It is important to note that there is an obvious selection bias for geriatric patients treated in the context of clinical research because patients that participate are typically fit patients who meet the multiple inclusion/exclusion criteria. Outcomes are not likely to be good in clinical practice.

It is generally felt that all patients with AML who achieve CR are destined to relapse at some point if the response is not consolidated with additional cycles of chemotherapy. Unfortunately, there is no proven standard of care for postremission consolidation in elderly patients at this time.[18,19,26] Whereas younger patients benefit from consolidation strategies that include HiDAC, randomized data to support HiDAC consolidation in elderly patients is lacking yet often administered (1–2 cycles, dose reduced for age) in clinical practice. This practice is based on the observation that in studies that have included geriatric patients with AML, the only long-term survivors are those that go on to receive postremission consolidation.[18] Consolidation and maintenance strategies with novel agents and those that include nonmyeloablative allogeneic transplantation represent exciting areas of current clinical investigation.[27–29] In terms of allogeneic transplantation, in the small subset of fit elderly patients who achieve a complete response and have a suitable available donor, stem cell transplantation can offer the potential for long-term disease-free survival with an acceptable treatment-related mortality.[30–32]

A major challenge in terms of risk stratification in elderly patients with AML is the determination of the relative importance of the various reported clinical and biological risk factors. Several models, which include clinical factors and cytogenetics, have been proposed and validated to help in this regard.[33–35] Patients deemed at "high risk" for failure with standard therapies should be spared the toxicity of traditional remission induction, as it has minimal if any long-term clinical benefit. It is reasonable for those patients to consider alternative less-intensive treatment approaches, supportive care measures and palliative options.[27,36]

Treatment options for unfit patients with AML remain limited at this time. A standard approach in Europe is to administer low-dose subcutaneous cytarabine (LDAC) in the office or home setting. This practice is based on the results of the AML 14 study, which included 212 patients (78% were age >70) who were not candidates for intensive therapy and who received either supportive care, including transfusions, antibiotics, hydroxyurea for white blood cell count control (1% CR rate), or supportive care and LDAC (18% CR rate). For the subset of LDAC responders, the median survival was 1.5 years (vs 2 months).[37] More recently, elderly patients unfit to receive standard therapy are receiving treatment in the form of a novel class of agents termed *DNA methyltransferase inhibitors* (DNMT) either as induction or in consolidation. There are currently 2 DNMT approved by the US Food and Drug Administration (FDA) for the treatment of myelodysplastic syndrome, decitabine and azacitidine. Both agents have shown promising activity in patients with AML.[38] Responses appear to be durable in patients with poor-risk cytogenetic profiles, something not observed in high-risk patients treated with low-dose cytarabine. Recently, Fenaux and coworkers[39] compared azacitidine versus investigator's choice of therapy (3+7, LDAC, or supportive care) in 358 patients with high-risk MDS or AML (32%). In that series, patients (MDS and AML) who received azacitidine had a statistically significantly improved overall survival compared with those who received investigator's choice (median, 24.5 vs

---

Box 1
Promising novel agents in AML

- DNA methyltransferase inhibitors (azacitidine, decitabine)[39]
- Histone deacetylase inhibitors[40–42]
- Purine nucleoside analogues (clofarabine, sapacitabine)[2,43]
- Sulfonylhydrazine alkalating agent (Larustine)
- Mammalian target of rapamycin inhibitors[44,45]
- Novel topoisomerase II inhibitors (voreloxin)[46–48]
- Fms-like tyrosine kinase 3 (FLT3) inhibitors[49]
- Angiogenesis inhibition/microenvironment (Lenalidomide)[50]

---

15 months).[39] Similar rates and duration of response have been observed when patients with AML are treated with decitabine as an induction agent.[38] A partial list of promising agents being studied in patients with AML who are not candidates for standard remission induction strategies are listed in **Box 1**.

Acute Lymphoblastic Leukemia

In terms of incidence, acute lymphoblastic leukemia (ALL) is far less common than AML in adults (1.7 per 100,000 men and women per year, SEER). Like AML, ALL is a disease with a median age of diagnosis in the sixth decade of life in adults; thus, many patients with ALL are within the geriatric patient population. Increased age is an important adverse prognostic feature of ALL and is most likely associated with the presence of clinical host poor prognostic factors (ie, comorbid conditions, intolerability of chemotherapy, poor nutritional status, medication interactions that may decrease chemotherapy efficacy, increased risk of life-threatening infections) as well as leukemia-related poor prognostic factors (higher proportion of Philadelphia Ph[+] chromosome positive disease, complex karyotypes, high white blood cell count at diagnosis, presence of aberrant myeloid markers, B-cell immunophenotype).[51]

Therapy

In adults, there is no universally accepted treatment approach for remission induction; however, most oncologists utilize various induction strategies that contain anthracyclines, vinca alkaloids, L-asparaginase, cytarabine, methotrexate, central nervous system (CNS) prophylaxis, and prolonged exposure to steroids (prednisone or dexamethasone). It should be noted that there is extremely limited data on efficacy and toxicity of standard approaches in geriatric patients.[52–56] Most of the major trials published in adult ALL over the previous decade have excluded patients older than 60 years.

In the elderly, rates of response (and durability of response) using traditional approaches reserved for younger adults and pediatric patients are significantly lower. For those who achieve a CR, relapse is the expectation for the majority of patients, regardless of the specific treatment approach. For example, all adult patients treated with the Hyper-CVAD regimen, have a 5-year overall survival rate (OS) of 38%. treatment related mortality increases dramatically with patients (15% for patients $\geq$ 60 years vs 2% for patients <60 years). Age 45 years and older was found to be an adverse prognostic factor in patients treated with Hyper-CVAD.[56] Patients treated with the CALGB regimen had a 9% risk of death during induction. Rates of remission were significantly decreased in patients older than 60 years (39%) versus patients age 35 to 59 (85%).[54] The complications of such approaches (more pronounced in geriatric patients) include increased rates of infection, thrombotic events, pancreatitis, hepatic insufficiency, neurotoxicity, bleeding events, avascular necrosis, and muscle wasting.[51,57,58]

A major advancement in ALL therapy has been the addition of tyrosine kinase inhibitors (TKI) such as imatinib or dasatinib to cytotoxic chemotherapy for ALL patients with the Ph+ chromosome t(9;22), a known poor risk feature and the most common chromosome abnormality in adult patients with ALL. The addition of a TKI (which inhibits the BCR-ABL fusion protein) to cytotoxic chemotherapy has led to CR rates in excess of 90%.[59–62] Recently, Ravandi and colleagues[63] reported their experience with the TKI dasatinib combined with Hyper-CVAD followed by dasatinib containing maintenance schedule in 35 patients (upper age was 79 years). In this series, a proportion of patients achieving CR was 94%, and the estimated 2-year survival rate was 64%.[63] Additionally, TKI therapies (imatinib, dasatinib) have shown impressive activity when administered without cytotoxic chemotherapy.[64,65] In the era of TKI therapy in Ph(+) ALL 2 questions remain to be answered: (1) is there a subset of patients with Ph(+) ALL with an available donor who should not undergo stem cell transplantation in CR1? and (2) for older patients with ALL, can cytotoxic chemotherapy doses be attenuated or even eliminated in the setting of TKI therapy without compromising outcomes?

ALL patients who achieve CR are generally recommended to receive prolonged treatment protocols that include consolidation, intensification, and maintenance therapy (generally administered over a period of 24+ months) or allogeneic stem cell transplantation (high-risk disease such as Ph+ or t(4;11)+ or all younger adult patients with standard-risk disease and a suitable sibling donor).[52,66,67] Because allografting with a myeloablative regimen is prohibitive (unacceptably high treatment-related mortality) in the geriatric patient population, newer methods that utilize less intensive conditioning regimens (termed *nonmyeloablative* or *reduced intensity*) are being studied in adult ALL.[68,69] Retrospective series from the Center for International Blood and Marrow Transplant Research and European Group for Blood and Marrow Transplantation suggest a 30% to 40% long-term survival rate using these techniques in highly selected patients in CR at the time of transplantation.[70]

Upon relapse, ALL is almost universally fatal, with an approximately 5% to 7% long-term disease-free survival rate reported and diminished rates (approximately 20%–30%) of second CR regardless of the salvage option used.[71,72] Patients with relapsed ALL are ideal candidates for consideration for clinical trial participation, as no standard of care exists. Promising agents being tested in relapsed/refractory ALL are listed in **Box 2**. For those who are able to obtain a second remission, candidacy for nonmyeloablative allogeneic transplantation should be considered. For the subset of patients who achieve a second CR, long-term survivors have been reported with reduced intensity allogeneic transplantation.[69]

Conclusion

Not all elderly patients with acute leukemia are destined to succumb to their disease, and careful consideration by the evaluating physician should incorporate and consider known risk factors with an aim to:

1. Identify the minority of patients who may benefit from standard approaches traditionally reserved for younger patients and implement therapy promptly

---

Box 2
Promising novel agents/potential pathways to target in ALL

- Liposomal formulation of traditional chemotherapy (vincristine/marqibo, novel liposomal anthracycline formulations)[70]
- BCR ABL TKI (imatinib, dasatinib)[64,65]
- New nucleoside analogues (clofarabine, nelarabine)[73–75]
- PNP inhibitors (forodesine)[75]
- Monoclonal antibodies (rituximab CD20, ofatumumab CD20, epratuzumab CD22, alemtuzumab CD52)[76–81]
- Immunoconjugates (Inotuzumab ozogamicin CD22)[82]
- Mammalian target of rapamycin inhibitors[83–88]
- Notch 1 inhibition (T-cell ALL)[89]
- Cyclin-dependant kinase inhibitors (Flavopiridol)[90–93]

---

2. Identify patients who are not candidates (based on clinical or biological risk factors) for intensive approaches to minimize treatment-related morbidity and mortality with consideration of alternative less-intensive therapies hopefully in the context of clinical research.
3. Identify patients who are not treatment candidates and discuss management strategies early on with a focus on supportive care, palliative medicine, and end-of-life discussions.

LYMPHOMA MANAGEMENT IN GERIATRIC MEDICINE

Lymphoma is the sixth most common malignancy in the United States. As per SEER data, it is estimated that 74,030 men and women (40,050 men and 33,980 women) will have lymphoma diagnosed, and 21,530 men and women will die of non-Hodgkin lymphoma (NHL) in 2010[1] (NCI's SEER Cancer Statistics Review).

Epidemiology

NHL is disease of elderly. The incidence of NHL is age dependent and increases dramatically with age. While incident rate for all NHL is 19.7 per 100,000 adults ages 20 to 64, it increases to 144 per 100,000 for ages 65 and older. NHL is also becoming more common; its incidence increased nearly 84% from the mid-1970s to 2010. From 2004 to 2008, the median age for diagnosis of lymphoma was 64 years of age.[3] Approximately 18.5% of the cases were diagnosed between ages 55 and 64; 20.4% between ages 65 and 74; 21.1% between ages 75 and 84; and 8.2% at 85+ years of age, bringing it a total of 68.2% of all cases of lymphoma diagnosed in people older than 55 years. From 2003 to 2007, the median age for death from lymphoma was 75 years.[4] Approximately 14.0% died between the ages of 55 and 64; 22.0% between 65 and 74; 33.1% between 75 and 84; and 17.7% at 85+ years, with a total of 86.8% of all lymphoma deaths occurring in people older 55 years. These rates are based on patients who died in 2003 to 2007 in the United States.

World Health Organization's (WHO) classification of tumors of hematopoietic and lymphoid tissues recognizes more than 30 different types of B and T cell lymphomas, based on clinical, histologic, immunophenotypic, and molecular biology features.

Diffuse large B-cell lymphoma, followed by follicular center cell lymphoma, is the most common in elderly adults (**Boxes 3** and **4**).

Some subtypes are seen exclusively in the elderly, such as primary cutaneous diffuse large B-cell lymphoma (DLBCL) leg type, Epstein-Barr virus (EBV)-positive DLBCL of elderly, whereas primary mediastinal DLBCL is rarely seen in that age group. **Table 1** represents incidence rates comparison between younger and elderly adults.

In the northern United States and Europe, the number of people older than 65 is increasing, and by 2030 they will be prevalent by number. The same trend is likely to occur in developing countries; as the quality of life improves, the number of children per family usually declines and longevity improves. Together with increasing incidence of NHL in the aging population, we can expect an increase in the number of lymphoma cases in the elderly.

Geriatric Assessment

What is the definition of elderly? Definitions derived from clinical research define elderly as 65 and older. Very elderly is 80 and older. Age influences the approach to treatment as it impacts a patient's ability to tolerate standard therapies that are typically recommended for younger patients. The majority of patients will present in the seventh decade of life.

Although decision making is much more straightforward in young patients, as treatment is generally administered with curative intent with the potential for substantial gains in quality-of-life years, treatment decisions are much more nuanced in the elderly. Data from clinical research are very limited because older patients are underrepresented in clinical trials.[94] Treatment decisions should be based on goals (curative, long-term remission, palliation), and take into account the frailty of the patient.

There are some unique circumstances in the treatment of elderly patients. Low normal physiologic parameters of healthy elderly, such as decreased hematopoietic and immunologic reserve, decreased detoxifying ability of the liver, and decreased glomerular filtration rate increases the toxicity of therapeutic drugs. Malnutrition, comorbidity, dependence, polypharmacy, and cognitive dysfunction are more likely to be present in elderly. Cultural and religious beliefs often impact patient choices more so than in younger patients. Some elders are concerned that receiving chemotherapy may impact family dynamics and place a burden on the family, thus, skewing their decision to pursue treatment options. Fixed income, lack of transportation, high cost of prescription medications, and a lack of family support are just few examples. Although patients with early dementia can navigate their daily routines, they have difficulties adjusting to new situations, making it difficult for them to adhere to multiple new medications (which are part of supportive measures during chemotherapy) and maintaining adequate hydration and nutrition during chemotherapy.

Routine history and physical, as done in busy practice, will not uncover important factors relevant to the success of treatment. Recoding an ECOG performance status and use of age-specific assessment tools are mandatory in elderly patients[95] to help judge a patient's candidacy for chemotherapy. To assist medical oncologists in developing an appropriate personalized treatment strategy and to identify potential remediable conditions, multiple geriatric assessment tools have been developed. They include formal cognitive, nutritional, functional, and social support status assessments.

The International Society of Geriatric Oncology has published Web-based comprehensive geriatric assessment (CGA) guidelines that can be accessed on line. CGA

Box 3
WHO 2008: the mature B-cell neoplasms

- Chronic lymphocytic leukemia/small lymphocytic lymphoma
- B-cell prolymphocytic leukemia
- Splenic marginal zone lymphoma
- Hairy cell leukemia
- *Splenic lymphoma/leukemia, unclassifiable*
- *Splenic diffuse red pulp small B-cell lymphoma[a]*
- *Hairy cell leukemia variant[a]*
- Lymphoplasmacytic lymphoma
- Waldenström macroglobulinemia
- Heavy chain diseases
- Alpha heavy chain disease
- Gamma heavy chain disease
- Mu heavy chain disease
- Plasma cell myeloma
- Solitary plasmacytoma of bone
- Extraosseous plasmacytoma
- Extranodal marginal zone B-cell lymphoma of mucosa-associated
- lymphoid tissue (MALT lymphoma)
- Nodal marginal zone B-cell lymphoma (MZL)
- *Pediatric type nodal MZL*
- Follicular lymphoma
- *Pediatric-type follicular lymphoma*
- Primary cutaneous follicle center lymphoma
- Mantle cell lymphoma
- DLBCL not otherwise specified
- T cell/histiocyte rich large B-cell lymphoma
- *DLBCL associated with chronic inflammation*
- *Epstein-Barr virus (EBV)[+] DLBCL of the elderly*
- Lymphomatoid granulomatosis
- Primary mediastinal (thymic) large B-cell lymphoma
- Intravascular large B-cell lymphoma
- *Primary cutaneous DLBCL, leg type*
- ALK[+] large B-cell lymphoma
- Plasmablastic lymphoma
- Primary effusion lymphoma
- *Large B-cell lymphoma arising in HHV8-associated multicentric Castleman disease*
- Burkitt lymphoma

- *B-cell lymphoma, unclassifiable, with features intermediate between diffuse large B-cell lymphoma and Burkitt lymphoma*
- B-cell lymphoma, unclassifiable, with features intermediate between diffuse large B-cell
- lymphoma and classical Hodgkin lymphoma
- **Hodgkin lymphoma**
- Nodular lymphocyte-predominant Hodgkin lymphoma
- Classical Hodgkin lymphoma
- Nodular sclerosis classical Hodgkin lymphoma
- Lymphocyte-rich classical Hodgkin lymphoma
- Mixed cellularity classical Hodgkin lymphoma
- Lymphocyte-depleted classical Hodgkin lymphoma

[a]These represent provisional entities or provisional subtypes of other neoplasms.

Diseases shown in italics are newly included in the 2008 WHO classification.

is time consuming and may not be feasible in a busy oncology practice. VES-13 (Vulnerable Elders Survey) is a less time-consuming tool that can identify patients for more formal evaluation with CGA.[96] Comorbidities and polypharmacy are associated with worse outcomes, as it was shown by Charlson and colleagues.[97] Cumulative Illness Rating Scale measures comorbidities.[98] Several practical geriatric assessment tools were developed and evaluated that can be used in the oncology practice. They involve a self-administered questionnaire as well as several functional tests (timed up and go, handgrip, gait and balance test).[99,100]

Risk Stratification

Many types of lymphoma are potentially curable, and most can be controlled with chemotherapy with palliative intent. The dilemma in the elderly patient population is deciding which patients are candidates for standard dose therapies and which patients are likely to suffer treatment-related morbidity and mortality. Sometimes a decision is made to treat patients using attenuated doses/schedules of chemotherapy; unfortunately, there is limited information as to how such modifications can impact efficacy.

Evens and coworkers[101] described the experience of 4 Chicago centers in treating 150 very elderly (older than 80 years) patients from 1999 until 2009. The presence of geriatric syndrome, Cumulative Illness Rating Scale for Geriatrics, and preservation of activity of daily living (ADL) were used to assess the "fitness" of the patients. Half of the patients had aggressive NHL and half-indolent NHL. Eighty-four percent of the patients with aggressive NHL had received at least 1 cycle of rituximab-containing chemotherapy, whereas only 35% patients received rituximab-containing chemotherapy. With 40-month median follow-up, 3-year event-free survival (EFS) and OS for all patients were 43.8% and 70.3%, respectively. Among aggressive NHL, 3-year EFS and OS were 55% and 64%, whereas for indolent NHL (n = 76), the 3-year EFS and OS were 34% and 77%, respectively. The strongest factors predicting survival in univariate analyses were failure to respond to initial therapy, unfit patient, loss of ADL, presence of geriatric syndrome, and low albumin level. The presence of diabetes as a comorbidity also negatively influenced outcomes. Utilizing CGA in addition to international prognostic index (IPI) score should become routine in oncology practice.

Box 4
WHO 2008: the mature T-cell and natural killer cell neoplasms

- T-cell prolymphocytic leukemia
- T-cell large granular lymphocytic leukemia
- Chronic lymphoproliferative disorder of natural killer cells[a]
- Aggressive natural killer cell leukemia
- *Systemic EBV+ T-cell lymphoproliferative disease of childhood(associated with chronic active EBV infection)*
- *Hydroa vacciniforme-like lymphoma*
- Adult T-cell leukemia/lymphoma
- Extranodal natural killer/T cell lymphoma, nasal type
- Enteropathy-*associated* T-cell lymphoma
- Hepatosplenic T-cell lymphoma
- Subcutaneous panniculitislike T-cell lymphoma
- Mycosis fungoides
- Sézary syndrome
- Primary cutaneous CD30[+] T-cell lymphoproliferative disorder
- Lymphomatoid papulosis
- Primary cutaneous anaplastic large-cell lymphoma
- *Primary cutaneous aggressive epidermotropic CD8+ cytotoxic T-cell lymphoma[a]*
- *Primary cutaneous gamma-delta T-cell lymphoma*
- *Primary cutaneous small/medium CD4+ T-cell lymphoma[a]*
- Peripheral T-cell lymphoma, not otherwise specified
- Angioimmunoblastic T-cell lymphoma
- Anaplastic large cell lymphoma, ALK[+]
- *Anaplastic large cell lymphoma, ALK–[a]*

[a]These represent provisional entities or provisional subtypes of other neoplasms.

Diseases shown in italics are newly included in the 2008 WHO classification.

Lymphoma Subtypes: Geriatric-Related Issues

Diffuse large B-cell lymphoma

DLBCL is a very heterogeneous disease based on the variety observed in terms of morphology, immunohistochemistry, clinical behavior, and gene-expression profiling. DLBCL can arise de novo or by transformation from low-grade B-cell lymphoma. Transformed DLBCL has much worse prognosis.

The cell of origin of DLBCL can be a germinal or postgerminal mature B cell. Pathogenesis of DLBCL is a multistep process, which involves overexpression of some and silencing of other genes. Using gene expression microarray technology, 3 subtypes of DLBCL were recognized: germinal center B-cell–like (GCB), activated B-cell–like (ABC), and non–otherwise-specified type 3.[102] The GCB DLBCL has a gene expression profile characteristic of normal germinal center B cells. The ABC

Table 1
Incidence rates of selected NHL subtypes, all races, both sexes, 2001–2008

Subtypes	Ages 20–64		Ages 65+	
	Rate	Count	Rate	Count
Hodgkin	3.3	12013	4.2	2962
NHL	19.7	74120	144.8	101501
Precursor non-Hodgkin lymphoma, B cell	0.6	2160	1.0	683
Mature B-cell NHL	16.5	62021	128.2	89840
Chronic/small lymphocytic leukemia/lymphoma	2.8	10654	31.7	22,281
DLBCL	4.7	17644	32.2	22628
Follicular lymphoma	3.0	11,401	15.1	10560
Non-Hodgkin lymphoma, T cell	1.7	6,358	6.8	4721
Precursor NHL, T cell	0.2	655	0.2	107
Mature Non-Hodgkin lymphoma, T cell	1.5	5,635	6.5	4,549
Peripheral T-cell lymphoma	0.9	3413	4.4	3068

Incidence per 100,000.
Adapted from SEER Cancer Statistics.

DLBCL has a gene expression profile similar to that of postgerminal center-activated B cells. ABC DLBCLs have high expression and constitutive activity of the nuclear factor kappa B (NF-KB) complex involved in the B-cell receptor (BCR) signaling pathway.[102] ABC DLBCLs carry mutations in multiple genes that activate NF-KB, including CARD11, TRAF2, and TRAF5.[103] Chronic active signaling of BCR is important in the survival of ABC DLBCL. The survival of ABC DLBCLs without CARD11 mutations appears to be dependent on the expression of another BCR signaling component known as *Bruton's tyrosine kinase* (BTK).[104] The Shipp group identified 3 subtypes of DLBCL using molecular profiling as "oxidative phosphorylation," "B-cell receptor/proliferation," and "host response."[105] Commonly overexpressed proteins in DLBCL are BCL-6, p53, and BCL-2.

GCB has overall survival advantage of almost 20% over ABC.[102] Rational treatment development based on subtypes of DLBCL is an active area of translational research. Two promising agents, which are currently in clinical trials, are inhibitors of SYK kinase and the Bruton tyrosine kinase—both of which are components of BCR signaling pathway that include multiple players. Unfortunately, microarray gene expression profile continues to be research domain for subclassification of DLBCL based on cell of origin. Reliable surrogate markers to identify GCB versus non-GCB DLBCL in clinical practice need to be developed. Several algorithms based on immunohistochemical stains of paraffin sections were developed. CD10 expression, BCL-2, bcl-6, foxP1, LMO1, and MUM1 are several markers. The most commonly used in clinical practice is Han's model.[106]

Clinical Presentation

The majority of the patients present with an advanced stage. Lymphadenopathy is usually not painful, and an invasion of adjacent organs rarely occurs that explains why DLBCL frequently gets detected at advanced stage. B symptoms—drenching night sweats, weight loss more than 10% of the body weight, and fevers—can occur in up to 30% of the patients. Although typically DLBCL presents with lymphadenopathy, it can involve virtually any tissue: bone marrow, liver, lungs, skin, gastrointestinal tract, CNS, bone, testes, and breast.

Clinical diagnosis and evaluation should include a comprehensive physical examination; imaging with a computed tomography scan (CT) of the chest, abdomen, and pelvis; and a bone marrow biopsy. Evaluation of functional status with echocardiogram, pulmonary function test, and CGA is important. A positron emission tomography (PET) scan during the initial evaluation has become common practice, although evidence-based data are lacking. The PET scan can be particularly useful in evaluating early-stage disease—treatment decisions may be changed in the case of upstaging.

A diagnostic biopsy should be based on an adequate sample—core needle biopsy or incisional/excisional biopsy of the affected lymph node. It is very important that a hematopathologist evaluates the specimen. An immunohistologic staining to assign DLBCL to GCB or non-GCB subtypes, evaluation Ki-67 index, EBV expression, and c-myc overexpression are all important prognostic markers that will affect decision making and prognosis.[106–108] DLBCL usually expresses pan-B-cell antigens such as CD19, 20, 22, and 79a and PAX5. Proliferation marker Ki-67 is usually expressed at 40% to 60%; highly proliferative tumors with Ki-67 greater than 80%, by some reports, have worse prognosis when treated with standard Rituximab, Cyclophosphamide, Hydroxydoxorubicin, Oncovin, Prednisone (R-CHOP).

The IPI is calculated after complete restaging. Taking into account certain clinical parameters (known risk factors), which are associated with inferior outcomes, separate prognostic subgroups can be distinguished according to IPI: low and low intermediate and intermediate-high and high-risk groups. Validity of the index has not changed after addition of Rituximab to treatment plan. Overall survival rates range from 90% at 3 years for low IPI to 60% for high IPI.[109]

Elderly patients can be divided into fit and frail and very elderly (older than 85).[110] Based on IPI and molecular markers, favorable/low stage and unfavorable/advanced stage categories are separated. The favorable/low category will include patients with stage I and II, no bulky disease, and no risk factors except age. The unfavorable/advanced group include advanced stage (III and IV) and one more risk factor.

Clinical judgment alone may not be adequate to identify "fit" patients for aggressive chemotherapy. In an Italian study,[111] patients (n = 88) older than 65 were stratified into "fit" or "frail" based on CGA. The treatment plan was based on clinical judgment only. Half of the patients were determined to be "fit" by clinical judgment, with half of the "fit" group belonging to "frail" based on CGA. Curiously, CGA-"frail" patients treated with aggressive chemotherapy fared as poorly as palliative care patients only.

The GOL (Gruppo Oncoematologica Linfomi)[112] based the treatment of DLBCL on CGA. In a prospective study from June 2000 to March 2006, 100 patients were treated. Patients with no comorbidities received CHOP or R-CHOP; for patients with moderate or severe cardiomyopathy, the use of anthracyclines was omitted (Cyclophosphamide, Vincristine, Prednisone [CVP] or Rituximab, Cyclophosphamide, Vincristine, Prednisone [R-CVP]); patients with diabetes didn't receive prednisone (Cyclophosphamide, Hydroxydoxorubicin, Oncovin (CHO), Cyclophosphamide, Epirubicin, Oncovin (ECO) or Rituximab, Cyclophosphamide, Hydroxydoxorubicin, Oncovin (R-CHO), Rituximab, Cyclophosphamide, Epirubicin, Oncovin [R-CEO]); patients with neuropathy received Cyclophosphamide, Hydroxydoxorubicin, Prednisone (CHP) or Rituximab, Cyclophosphamide, Hydroxydoxorubicin, Prednisone (R-CHP) or Cyclophosphamide, Epirubicin, Prednisone (CEP) or Rituximab, Cyclophosphamide, Epirubicin, Prednisone (R-CEP) (vincristine was omitted). The dosage of chemotherapy was decided according to the CGA: patients with a good score of CGA (ie, ADL = 6 and IADL >6) received full doses of CT; patients with an intermediate score (ADL = 5 and IADL >4) received 75% of the planned dose; patients with a poor score (ADL <5 and IADL <5) received 50% of the planned dose. Sixty-one percent of patients received full doses of CT; 25% received 75% of dose and 14% received 50% reduced dose; 86% of patients received anthracycline and 54% rituximab. The majority of the patients were able to receive an anthracycline-containing regimen, with only 14% receiving CVP or R-CVP. The 5-year OS, disease-free survival, and EFS were 58%, 78%, and 50%, respectively.

Six cycles of R-CHOP remains the standard of care in treating DLBCL. This practice was established by the Groupe d'Etude des Lymphomes de l'Adulte (GELA) group.[113] Long-term follow-up[114] confirmed sustainable benefit in overall survival at 5-year follow-up. There is no advantage in giving 8 cycles as used to be customary.[115] Radiotherapy to the sites of bulky disease does not give survival advantage to elderly patients who achieve CR or complete remission unconfirmed after six cycles of R-CHOP.[116] Maintenance with Rituximab after initial treatment with Rituximab–containing regimen is not beneficial.[117]

Adherence to dose density and intensity is very important: while 98% of patients in the RICOVER60 trial were able to receive full doses of chemotherapy, it does not necessarily transmit to community practice as per a nationwide survey of records of 4522 patients with aggressive lymphomas treated with R-CHOP–like regimens in 567 oncology practices. For 60% of patients older than 60, relative dose intensity was 85% or less.

Unfortunately, up 40% of patients treated for DLBCL will ultimately experience relapse. Two large prospective trials: PARMA and CORAL, have established autologous stem cell transplant rescue of relapsed DLBCL as standard of care in fit patients with responding disease. PARMA compared chemotherapy only salvage versus chemotherapy plus high-dose chemotherapy with autologous stem cell transplant (SCT) showing significant survival advantage (OS at 53% and 12% at 5 years, respectively).[118] CORAL straddled the pre-rituximab and rituximab era and compared 2 rituximab-containing salvage regimens (RICE and RDHAP) followed by high-dose chemotherapy with autologous stem cell transplant followed by rituximab maintenance.[119] The CORAL study corroborated PARMA data and identified a group of patients with minimal benefit from autologous SCT salvage—those who had relapse within 12 months after initial treatment, which included Rituximab. Their survival rate was only around 20%.

While fit patients are eligible for transplant, the majority of elderly patients with relapsed DLBCL will not be candidates for autologous stem cell transplant. Autologous and allogeneic stem cell transplant can be performed successfully in the elderly patient. Age alone should not prevent referral to a transplant program for evaluation.[120–124]

Elderly patients are much less likely to have a second chance at cure; approaches to identify "bad players" and develop front-line therapies for high-risk patients are important. Hamlin and colleagues[125] used a strategy of consolidating R-CHOP with radioimmunotherapy with yttrium-90 ibritumomab tiuxetan (RIT) in high IPI elderly patients. OS and progression-free survival (PFS) at 42 months for RIT-treated patients (n = 44 of 65 enrolled) was 83.5% and 74.5%, respectively, which is significantly higher than the historical rate of 60%. Zinzani and colleagues[126] reported a similar trial for CHOP (without Rituximab) followed by consolidation with RIT.

Aggressive lymphomas, such as Burkitt's, pose a particular challenge. CHOP has demonstrated quite poor outcomes, with OS being around 25%. High-dose regimens, such as McGrath (hyperfractionated cyclophosphamide, doxorubicin, vincristine alternating with ifosfamide, etoposide, and cytarabine) or HyperCVAD, improve cures rate to up to 70%. These regimens are unlikely to be tolerated by majority of elderly patients. However, a selected group of "fit" individuals will be cured with an aggressive approach. In our practice, we have treated patients up to age 75 with Hyper CVAD and modified McGrath with successful outcomes.

CNS Prophylaxis

Depending on the series, up to 20% of aggressive and intermediate lymphomas relapse in the CNS mainly as lymphomatous meningitis and rarely as parenchymal brain involvement. Risk factors are extranodal involvement, bone marrow involvement, and testicular and head and upper neck involvement. Standard practice used to be intrathecal administration of methotrexate or cytarabine with each cycle of systemic therapy. With incorporation of rituximab into treatment of DLBCL, the benefit of intrathecal prophylaxis is under doubt. As reported in RICOVER-60,[127] estimated 2-year incidence of CNS disease was 6.9% after CHOP-14 and 4.1% after R-CHOP. Patients treated with R-CHOP did not show benefit from intrathecal methotrexate. Rituximab appears to diminish the risk of CNS disease. In our practice, patients with aggressive NHL such as Burkitt's and immunoblastic and lymphoblastic lymphoma and with testicular involvement are still treated with prophylactic intrathecal chemotherapy.

EBV-Associated DLBCL of the Elderly

EBV is a herpes virus that infects the majority of humans in childhood and has tropism for lymphocytes. Its capacity to immortalize B and T lymphocytes is well known. Levels of EBV-infected lymphocytes are kept at less than 5% by T cells. As T-cell function declines with age, the risk of EBV-infected lymphocytes to transform to lymphoma increases. EBV-positive DLBCL of the elderly (previously known as senile EBV-positive DLBCL) is recognized by WHO as provisional entity. It was originally described by Oyama and colleagues.[128] Patients tend to be older, are more likely to present with high IPI, have extranodal involvement, have B symptoms, and have no known immunodeficiency. Most importantly, they have a poor prognosis—less than 2 years of median survival. Its incidence among Asian and Latin American patient ranges from 9% to 15% and increases with age.[108] The incidence of EBV-DLBCL appears to be much less common in the western world, although the number of patients in the series are relatively small.[129,130] It is not routine practice to screen for EBV in DLBCL, potentially minimizing true incidence.

The theory behind EBV DLBCL of the elderly is a combination of immunosenescence, which affects mainly cellular immunity, and particular human leucocyte antigen (HLA) phenotype (potentially explaining difference in incidence between Asian and Western populations). A histologic distinction of EBV DLBCL is that infiltration of the lymph node can be quite polymorphic, with large cell and Reed-Sternberg–like cells mixed with reactive cells such as plasma cells, histiocytes, and small benign lymphocytes. The cell of origin is considered to be of a postgerminal center lymphocyte. Immunophenotypically, malignant cells are positive for CD45, CD20, CD19, CD79a; PAX5, CD10, and bcl6—germinal center markers—are usually negative. Proliferation marker Ki-67 is high. Up to 50% of the cell may express activation marker CD30, usually present on activated T cells, some peripheral T cell lymphoma and Hodgkin lymphoma. EBV-related proteins, LMP1 and EBNA-2, are positive in 94% and 28% of cases.[129] Typical EBV latency pattern in this lymphoma is II or III. The most sensitive methodology to detect the presence of EBV is in situ hybridization for EBV-encoded RNA. Because of the rarity of the entity, prospective clinical trials specifically addressing treatment of EBV DLBCL of the elderly are lacking. The poor prognosis label also comes from data of chemotherapy given without Rituximab. Our current approach is to treat these patients as other elderly with DLBCL with R-CHOP.

Primary CNS DLBCL

Primary CNS lymphoma (PCNSL) is an extranodal lymphoma that involves the brain, spinal cord, leptomeninges, and intraocular sites. It rarely spreads outside of CNS. While some of PCNSL are low grade and T cell, the majority is DLBCL. The median age at presentation is in the fifth decade with an incidence that increases with age. Immunodeficiency plays an important role in the development of PCNSL; human immunodeficiency virus (HIV)-related PCNSL, which is 100% EVB driven has been recognized. The typical presentation is a solitary lesion in periventricular brain structures (thalamus, basal ganglia, corpus callosum). Up to 25% of patients will have leptomeningeal involvement. Primary leptomeningeal lymphoma is extremely rare. Primary ocular lymphoma is a PCNSL that involves posterior eye: retina, vitreous body, and choroid. Clinical symptoms depend on the area of the CNS involved: focal neurologic deficits, neuropsychiatric symptoms, seizures, and ocular symptoms. PCNSL is medical emergency, particularly when there are signs of increased intracranial pressure, as the condition may progress quickly to herniation. It is rapidly fatal if left untreated. Typically, the establishment of diagnosis is delayed because presenting symptoms are nonspecific. In elderly patients, change in behavior may be assumed to be depression or early dementia, thus, delaying diagnosis until more ominous neurologic symptoms develop. Any elderly patient with rapid onset of dementia should be evaluated for PCNSL.

The diagnosis is typically made by stereotactic needle brain biopsy. Surgical excision should be avoided, as there is no clinical benefit for surgical resection. Clinical evaluation, in addition to physical examination and history, should include magnetic resonance imaging with gadolinium of the brain and total spine and slit lamp ocular examination. Lumbar puncture should be performed unless signs of increased intracranial pressure are present. PCNSL has a unique appearance on gadolinium-enhanced magnetic resonance imaging. Systemic lymphoma must be ruled out with CT scans of the chest, abdomen, pelvis, or PET scan and bone marrow biopsy. Testicular ultrasound scan is recommended if physical examination findings suggest testicular mass, because testicular DLBCL can present with parenchymal brain lesion. HIV testing is always performed.[131]

Optimal treatment is not clear. Multiple prospective and retrospective studies evaluated different treatment options. High-dose methotrexate-based therapy with or without whole-brain radiation provides the best survival. Consolidation with whole-brain radiotherapy prolongs PFS but not the OS and carries a greater than 50% chance of debilitating neurologic side effects, such as intellectual decline, balance, and incontinence in elderly patients. It is now customary to defer use of whole-brain RT in elderly patients.

The majority of elderly patients will tolerate high-dose methotrexate.[132,133] The most feared side effect is acute renal failure leading to delayed clearance of methotrexate. Methotrexate is not dialyzable and excreted exclusively by the kidneys. Thorough evaluation of kidney function is mandatory. Twenty-four–hour urine collection to determine creatinine clearance rather than calculated creatinine clearance is preferred. A decrease in glomerular filtration rate is not sole exclusion for using high dose methotrexate (HDMTX).[134]

The addition of other chemotherapeutic agents to high-dose methotrexate is unlikely to add to efficacy to the regimen but will increase toxicity. Adding cytarabine to methotrexate may improve PFS. High-dose cytarabine carries a high risk of hematologic toxicity and life-threatening infectious complications, particularly in patients older than 75 years.[135]

The combination of rituximab, HDMTX, and temozolomide was evaluated in a large prospective study and is a reasonable option in elderly.[136] Overall response rate ranged from 44% to 60%, and median OS is in the range of 32 months. Treatment options at relapse include using high-dose methotrexate. Other agents, such as temozolomide in combination with rituximab[137] and topotecan[138] have been studied and have some activity. Palliative radiation of the whole brain may be considered.

Hodgkin Lymphoma

Hodgkin lymphoma is considered a disease of children and young adults. However, Hodgkin lymphoma has a bimodal age distribution curve second to being in sixth decade. It represents about 10% of all lymphomas. It typically presents as painless lymphadenopathy. Frequently, patients may have pruritus, rashes, night sweats, fevers, and weight loss for prolonged periods before lymphadenopathy becomes apparent.

The diagnosis is made by incisional biopsy. Core needle biopsy is utilized, particularly in difficult-to-access anatomic areas. Fine-needle aspiration has very low sensitivity and should be avoided. The hallmark cell of HD, the Reed-Sternberg cell, is usually found in a background of inflammatory cells. Reed-Sternberg cells express CD15, CD30, and HLA-DR and lack pan-B and pan-T cell antigens. Occasionally, RS cells may express CD20, which is B-cell marker. The cell of origin of HD was not known until fairly recently when using single-cell microdissection techniques, it was proven that HD originates from B lymphocyte.

Histologically, there are several subtypes: nodular sclerosis, mixed cellularity, lymphocyte rich, and lymphocyte depleted. Nodular sclerosis is the most predominant in young adults. Mixed cellularity, which is more likely to be associated with EBV, is more prevalent in the elderly. Lymphocyte-rich and lymphocyte-depleted subtypes are less common; lymphocyte-depleted HD is associated with worse prognosis and with immunodeficiency such as HIV. A separate entity of HD—lymphocyte-predominant nodular (nonclassical) HD—has been described. It behaves more like a low-grade lymphoma, and typically responds to rituximab-containing regimens as well as single-agent rituximab, as the malignant cells in lymphocyte predominant nodular Hodgkin lymphoma express CD20.

HD is a very curable disease. Treatment approaches used in elderly patients are similar to those for young adults: for early stage/low risk, abbreviated course of ABVD (Adriamycin, bleomycin, vinblastine, dacarbazine) followed by involved field radiation; for advanced stage, 6 cycles of ABVD. A major challenge is that tolerability of ABVD by elderly is poor. A significant proportion of elderly patients may not have adequate pulmonary function or cardiac reserve. A large retrospective analysis of the German Hodgkin Study Group database showed that elderly patients are much more likely to experience acute toxicity. Only 75% of patients as opposed to 91% of younger patients were able to complete chemotherapy as intended. Overall survival rate was only 65% at 5 years compared with 90% in patients less than 60.[139]

Worse outcomes transcend stage and risk factors as confirmed by HD8 trial, which studied early stage with or without unfavorable risk factors. Treatment was 4 cycles of ABVD followed by involved or extended field radiation. The radiation toxicity was significantly higher, with overall 5-year survival rate only 74% in patients older than 60 versus 94% in patients younger than 60. Extended field radiation was so poorly tolerated that recommendation was made against extended-field radiation therapy.[140]

To address the issue of poor tolerability of chemotherapy by elderly patients, German Hodgkin Lymphoma Study Group is conducting a phase II study of PVAG (prednisone, vinblastine, doxorubicin, gemcitabine) in patients between 60 and 75 years old. Preliminary results show that OS at 3 year is 66% and PFS is 58%. The regimen is much better tolerated.

A recent breakthrough in the treatment of relapsed HD is the approval of brentuximab vedotin (SGN-3) in relapsed refractory HD. Brentuximab Vedotin is a drug-antibody conjugate linking CD30 antibody with monomethyl auristatin. In the pivotal trial, the response rate was 75%. Data on OS and PFS are not yet available.[141] The drug is very well tolerated. A trial using SGN-35 in combination in with adriamycin, vinblastin, dacarbazine (omitting bleo) in front-line settings is ongoing.

The art of treating curable lymphomas such as HD and DLBCL is to avoid Pyrrhic victory: not to jeopardize efficacy of therapy while avoiding toxicity, which will negate the effect.

Low Grade Lymphomas

Follicular lymphoma (FL) is the second most common lymphoma, comprising approximately 20% of NHL in the United States and Western Europe. It is the most common low-grade lymphoma, presenting as 70% of all low-grade B-cell lymphomas.

Normal counterpart is a B-cell derived from the germinal center of the lymph node. The hallmark genetic mutation of FL is translocation of (14;18), which results in overexpression of B-cell leukemia/lymphoma 2 (BCL-2). BCL-2 is antiapoptotic protein. Multiple genetic events must happen before development of FCL. Interestingly, t(14;18) is present in small proportion of normal individuals.

Histologically, FL has nodular growth pattern preserving normal germinal centers. Several grades are recognized based on presence of centroblasts. Increased number centroblasts correlates with increased aggressiveness of FL. Grade I and II are considered low grade, whereas grade III is believed to behave as DLBCL. Grade III is divided into IIIa and IIIb. IIIa is considered to behave as indolent and IIIb aggressively. Unfortunately, variability between pathologists in assigning grade (particularly IIIa vs IIIb) is quite high.

Immunophenotypically, FL is usually CD10 positive, CD20 positive, or CD79a-positive and stains for intracytoplasmic BCL2. Clinically, it presents as painless adenopathy at the time of diagnosis and frequently involves bone marrow. B symptoms are uncommon. It frequently has a very indolent course; however, some patients relapse and progress within couple of years, whereas others may have asymptomatic disease for years. The Follicular Lymphoma International Prognostic Index (FLIPI) score and grade are important in predicting clinical behavior. Recently, the importance of the microenvironment was shown in several studies. Infiltration of the tumor by CD8 T cells was associated with longer survival. Up to 25% of disease may transform to aggressive lymphoma, which carries poor prognosis (**Table 2**).

PFS and OS at 5 years is 91%, 78%, and 52% for low, intermediate, and high FLIPI1, respectively. PFS at 3 years was 91%, 69%, and 51% for patients with low (0 factors), intermediate (1–2 factors), or high (3–5) FLIPI2, respectively.

FL carries favorable prognosis. The dogma of treatment used to be that it is incurable disease, and chemotherapy does not affect OS. With advent of rituximab, long-term data from SEER shows prolongation of OS in the rituximab era and hint at the possibility of cure.

Table 2
Two FLIPI versions

FLIPI1[142]	FLIPI2[143]
Age over 60	Age over 60
Ann Arbor stage III or IV	Bone marrow involvement
Hemoglobin level <12 g/dL	Hemoglobin level <12 g/dL
Number of involved nodal areas more than 4	Longest diameter of largest lymph node >6 cm
LDH greater than upper limit of normal	b2-microglobulin>ULN

The goal of treatment in the elderly should be achieving palliation of symptoms and long-term remissions with preservation of quality of life. The initial treatment depends on symptomatology. Watch and wait approach in asymptomatic patients is becoming less practiced. Watch and wait is quite reasonable in elderly asymptomatic patients.[144] Traditional indications to start treatment are presence of B symptoms, bone marrow failures (Hb <11g/dL, neutrophils <1500/mL, thrombocytes <100,000), large tumor burden, rapid progression, or disease-related symptomatology such as pain or splenic infarct. An intergroup trial comparing 3 arms: watch and wait, rituximab induction, and rituximab induction and maintenance is ongoing. Rituximab alone is a quite commonly used strategy in front-line and relapsed disease. Response rate for upfront therapy is around 70% with duration of response over a year.[145,146]

If rapid debulking is required, combination immunochemotherapy is the usual approach. Several regimens are appropriate- R-CHOP, R-CVP, or R-Bendamustine.[147] A recent trial presented in abstract form comparing R-CHOP and R-bendamustine (BR) showed similar results with less toxicity for BR. Publication is being awaited.[148]

Whether to give maintenance rituximab after induction or just observe is still an area of contention, although more evidence is accumulating in favor of maintenance. The latest trial reported (PRIMA) suggests significant advantage of maintenance rituximab in patients treated with R-chemotherapy (most patients received R-CHOP) in the front-line setting.[149]

RIT using antibodies to CD20 conjugated to radioactive Iodine or Yttrium is highly active in front-line settings in FL and can be particularly convenient in elderly patients. Consolidation with RIT (Yttrium) after original treatment with CHOP was studied (FIT study) with a high rate of partial response to complete response conversion and increased PFS (36 months vs 13 months) was shown.[150] A downside of the trial is that rituximab was not used as part of the induction regimen. Preliminary results of an intergroup trial presented as abstract at ASH 2010 did not find advantage in adding Bexxar (anti-CD20 antibody linked to Iodine121) to R-CHOP. Final results are awaited.

Relapsed patients may be retreated with rituximab alone, immunochemotherapy, or RIT, and selected patients may benefit from autologous or allogeneic transplant. Enrollment in clinical trials should be considered.

New therapeutics targeting molecular pathways and microenvironment are being developed including PI3delta kinase inhibitor, BTK inhibitor, lenalidomide, Anti-CD23 antibodies (epratuzumab), novel anti-CD20 antibodies (ofatumumab, veltuzumab GA 101), drug-antibody conjugates (inotuzumab ozogamicin), and Velcade.

There are still many unanswered questions in management of FL, and more clinical trials with large numbers of patients enrolled are needed.

MULTIPLE MYELOMA MANAGEMENT IN THE GERIATRIC MEDICINE
Epidemiology and Myeloma Statistics

Plasma cell dyscrasias are a heterogeneous group of disorders characterized by the neoplastic proliferation of plasma cells. Plasma cells are terminally differentiated B lymphocytes whose typical function is the production of antibody proteins. Multiple myeloma (MM) is defined by the presence of neoplastic plasma cells that directly lead to end-organ dysfunction in the form of anemia, renal failure, lytic bone disease, or hypercalcemia.

MM represents approximately 10% of all hematologic neoplasms and 1% of all cancer deaths. Last year 20,180 people had MM diagnosed and 10,650 died of the disease.[151] The median age at onset is 66 years with only 2% of patients younger than 40 years at diagnosis.[152] The management of MM in the geriatric population has a variety of unique concerns. One of the primary branch points in the decision tree for the management of newly diagnosed patients relates to eligibility for high-dose therapy and autologous stem cell transplantation. Additional factors affecting decision making include the presence of comorbid conditions and their subsequent association with polypharmacy.

Monoclonal Gammopathy of Undetermined Significance and Smoldering Myeloma

With the gradual aging of the general population, and the increase in prevalence of plasma cell dyscrasias with advancing age, it is anticipated that the diagnoses of these disorders will continue to increase over time. They often are found through laboratory and imaging workup for conditions such as anemia, renal insufficiency, and back pain. Given the sensitivity of current testing modalities, often these problems are discovered before they have (or will) manifest themselves clinically. MGUS refers to a low-burden disease state characterized by low levels of circulating monoclonal protein (<3 g/dL) as well as low levels of bone marrow infiltration of plasma cells (<10%) in concert with an absence of end-organ dysfunction attributable to the gammopathy. In a population-based study in Olmstead County, Minnesota, it was found that the average age for diagnosis of MGUS was 72, with 59% of patients being over the age of 70. With an overall prevalence of 5.3% of people aged 70 and older and 7.5% of people over the age of 85, the condition is quite common.[153]

MGUS carries with it a risk of progression to symptomatic neoplasm (eg, myeloma, lymphoma) of approximately 1% per year. Independent risk factors for risk of progression include abnormal free light chain ratio, immunoglobulin subtype (non–immunoglobulin G denotes a higher risk), and size of the M protein (>1.5 g/dL). Those with all 3 adverse factors have a risk of progression at 20 years of 58% compared with 37%, 21%, and 5% for 2, 1 and 0 risk factors, respectively.[154] The standard of care remains laboratory disease assessment on an every 6- to 12-month basis.

Smoldering (asymptomatic) MM represents a higher disease burden state with either bone marrow plasmacytosis greater than 10% or serum M protein >3.0 g/dL with the continued absence of gammopathy attributable end-organ dysfunction. The average age of diagnosis of this disorder ranges between 65 and 70 years of age and is felt to comprise approximately 10% to 15% of all cases of multiple myeloma.[155]

Of particular concern regarding these entities, relating to elderly patients, is the notion of attribution of clinical and laboratory abnormalities. Implicit in the definitions of MGUS and smoldering MM are the notions of gammopathy-related organ dysfunction. Renal disease in the elderly population often stems from metabolic causes, such as hypertensive and diabetic nephropathy.

Table 3
Staging systems

Stage	Durie-Salmon	International Staging System
I	Hemoglobin >10 g/dL	Serum B2M <3.5 mg/L
	Serum Calcium <10.5 mg/dL	Serum Albumin ≥3.5 g/dL
	Bone radiograph, normal bone structure (scale 0), or solitary plasmacytoma only	
	Low M-spike: IgG <5 g/dL, IgA <3 g/dL	
	Urine light chain M-component <4 g/24h	
II	Not stage I or stage III	Not stage I or stage III
III	Hemoglobin <8.5 g/dL	
	Serum calcium >12 mg/dL	
	Advanced lytic bone lesions 9scale 3)	
	High M-spike: IgG >7g/dL, IgA >5g/dL	
	Urine light chain M-component > 12 g/24 h	Serum B2M >5.5 mg/L
	Subclassification	A: Serum creatinine <2.0 mg/dL
	B: Serum creatinine >2.0 mg/dL	

Anemia in the elderly may also present an issue. It is prudent to rule out the possibility of vitamin/mineral deficiencies such as iron, b12, and folate. Given the incidence of myelodysplastic syndromes in this patient population, as well as the limitations of peripheral blood testing, it may be somewhat difficult to rule out this diagnosis without a bone marrow aspiration and biopsy complete with cytogenetic evaluation. Careful history and physical examination (as well as serum ferritin) should be used to rule out anemia caused by chronic disease/inflammation.

Skeletal events must also be evaluated carefully given the incidence of osteoporosis in patients of this age group. Bone densitometry should be utilized and its results used in conjunction with disease burden assessments to determine the likely cause of any skeletal event or abnormality. In addition, other tumors (such as prostate carcinoma) may be associated with lytic bone disease and should be considered during the evaluation.

Staging and Risk Stratification

Staging and risk stratification for elderly patients with myeloma is no different from that of their younger cohorts. There are 2 staging systems that have been used to describe patients with MM: the Durie-Salmon[156] staging system and the International Staging System.[157] Although the staging systems do not offer guidance toward directing therapy, they do provide prognostic information; with higher stage connoting shorter predicted survival (**Table 3**).

With the advent of cytogenetic and FISH techniques, we are now able to delineate those with "higher-risk" disease. The currently accepted risk factors are listed in **Table 4**.[158]

The feeling from the consensus paper is that those with high-risk disease should be treated initially with a bortezomib-based regimen, whereas those with standard risk can be treated either with a lenalidomide- or bortezomib-based therapy. The rationale behind this stems from the fact that bortezomib may overcome some of the adverse effects of high-risk genetics, particularly in cases of t(4;14).

Table 4
Risk stratification

High Risk	Standard Risk
Del 17p	Hyperdiploidy
T(4;14)	T(11;14)
T(14;16)	T(6;14)
Del 13q[a]	
Hypodiploidy	
Plasma Cell Labeling Index ≥3%	

[a] Del 13q denotes high-risk when appreciated on routine cytogenetics and not solely by FISH.

Transplantation in the Elderly

With more than 37% of newly diagnosed patients aged 75 years or older,[159] the presence of comorbid medical conditions in conjunction with relative declinations in performance status often lead to concerns for clinicians offering high-dose therapy to this patient population. It has been shown in multiple clinical trials that patients treated with high-dose therapy, followed by autologous stem cell rescue, have improved survival compared with matched cohorts receiving conventional-dose therapy (**Table 5**).[160]

After induction therapy, stem cell mobilization and collection can be achieved through 1 of 3 main approaches: (1) chemotherapy-stimulated mobilization (followed by growth factors), (2) growth factors alone, or (3) growth factors plus plerixafor a CXCR4 receptor antagonist. There are a variety of options for chemotherapy based mobilizing regimens, which are listed in **Table 6**. Intermediate dose cyclophosphamide is one of the more common approaches. The benefit of chemotherapy-based mobilization is multifaceted in terms of peripheral blood stem cell yield as well as the potential for antitumor effect.

Morris and colleagues[167] from the University of Arkansas discovered that advancing age was associated with an incremental decrease in CD34+ stem cell collection; however, the total yield was strongly correlated with mobilization regimen, length of prior therapy, and premobilization platelet count. Numerous studies have resulted in conflicting results regarding age as an independent predictor of stem cell yield. Chemotherapy-based mobilization regimens, in general,

Table 5
Demographics

Age Group	Percentage of People with MM	Percentage of People Who Died of MM
<20	0	0
20–34	0.5	0.1
35–44	3.3	1.2
45–54	12	6.3
55–64	21.6	16.3
65–74	26.5	26.2
75–84	26.4	34.4
>85	9.8	15.5

Table 6
Mobilizing regimens

Mobilizing Regimen	Regimen Details	Publication
C	Cyclophosphamide 4 g/m^2 or Cyclophosphamide 1.2 ->2 g/m^2	To et al, 1990[161] Jantunen et al, 2003[162]
CDEP	Cyclophosphamide 400 mg/m^2/d CIVI × 4 d Dexamethasone 40 mg/d × 4 d Etoposide 40 mg/m^2/d CIVI × 4 d Cisplatin 10 mg/m^2/day CIVI × 4 d	Lazzarino et al, 2001[163]
CVAD	Cyclophosphamide 500 mg/m^2/day × 4 d Vincristine 2 mg on day 1 Doxorubicin 50 mg/m^2/day on days 1 and 2 Dexamethasone 40 mg/d × 4 d	Majolino et al, 1995[164]
VAD	Vincristine 0.4 mg/d × 5 d Doxorubicin 9 mg/m^2/d × 5 d Dexamethasone 40 mg/d × 5 d	Lefrere et al, 2006[165]
VDT-PACE	Bortezomib 1.0 mg/m^2 days 1, 4, 8, 11 Thalidomide 200 mg/d days 1->4 Dexamethasone 40mg/day days 1->4 Cisplatin 10 mg/m^2/d days 1->4 Doxorubicin 10 mg/m^2/d days 1->4 Cyclophosphamide 400 mg/m^2/d days 1->4 Etoposide 40 mg/m^2/d days 1->4	Barlogie et al, 2007[166]

resulted in greater collection of CD34+ cells; however, this effect was lost on patients with longer duration of therapy before mobilization (>12 months) and platelet count <200 × 10^9/L. These results suggest that elderly patients, in particular, would benefit from early stem cell collection rather than collection late in their course of therapy. Toxicities seen in the chemotherapy-mobilized patients were statistically higher than those mobilized with growth factors alone and were mostly constitutional symptoms and neutropenic fever. In this study, no patient was unable to proceed toward high-dose therapy and transplant after mobilization with chemotherapy.

For more frail patients, in whom cytotoxic chemotherapy may be prohibitive, one has the option of mobilizing with growth factor support with or without Plerixafor. Plerixafor is a first-in-class small molecule that inhibits binding to the CXC chemokine receptor 4. It was originally studied as a potential therapy for HIV because of the virus' selective tropism for that receptor. The drug's ability to increase the circulating CD34+ cell count led to further study in the realm of hematopoietic stem cell transplantation. In a study by DiPersio and coworkers,[168] 54% of the patients treated with plerixafor (with concomitant granulocyte colony-stimulating factor) reached their target collection goal after 1 pheresis versus 56% of the patients treated with granulocyte colony-stimulating factor alone who required 4 sessions to achieve equivalent targets. Plerixafor is very well tolerated with the main toxicities being injection site reaction and gastrointestinal upset.

High-dose melphalan (MEL200) remains the standard approach for conditioning in eligible patients for autologous stem cell transplantation.[169] A recent article by Bashir and coworkers[170] evaluated the feasibility of this approach in patients older than 70 years. The standard dose (for younger patients) is 200 mg/m^2 given intravenously either in 1 day or divided across 2 days. Dose reductions have been used based on clinician's discretion. The overall response rate (CR+VGPR+PR) for MEL140,

---

Box 5
Therapeutic classes/pathways in myeloma

Steroids: Dexamethasone, Prednisone

Immunomodulatory (ImID): Thalidomide, Lenalidomide

Proteasome Inhibition (PI): Bortezomib

Alkylators: Melphalan, Cyclophosphamide

Other classic chemotherapeutics: Liposomal doxorubicin, etoposide

Histone Deacytlase Inhibition (HDACi): Vorinostat, Panobinostat

Monoclonal Antibodies: Elotuzumab (anti-CS1)

Mammalian target of Rapamycin (mTOR)

Hedgehog inhibitors

Akt/PI3K signaling pathways

MEL180, and MEL 200 are 88%, 90%, and 82%, respectively (the differences were not statistically significant).[170] The predictors of improved OS in these patients were timing of transplant (better outcome when performed in first remission as compared with relapsed disease) and disease status before transplant (>PR connotes better survival). Although there were increases in incidence of grade II–IV cardiac and gastrointestinal toxicity seen in escalating doses of melphalan, these differences were not statistically significant. In addition, the subgroup analysis between outcomes and morbidity/mortality of the 70 to 74 versus those ≥75 years of age showed no significant differences. The overall nonrelapse mortality rate was 3%. The conclusions from this publication are simply that age alone should not defer patients toward proceeding to high-dose therapy and autologous stem cell transplantation. This modality of therapy remains a viable treatment strategy for elderly patients with myeloma.

Induction Therapy in Transplant and Nontransplant Candidates

Once the diagnosis of symptomatic multiple myeloma is confirmed, the next step is the initiation of systemic therapy. The last 5 to 10 years have seen marked advancement in the development of novel therapies for this malignancy. There are a variety of 2-, 3-, and 4-drug regimens that are associated with overall response rates of greater than 90%. The decision of which drugs to utilize in the up-front setting should take into account several factors: (1) transplant eligibility, (2) performance status, (3) cytogenetic risk stratification, (4) comorbid conditions, (5) toxicity profile, and (6) renal function (**Box 5**).

Transplant eligibility is the key decision branch point in the management of newly diagnosed patients with multiple myeloma. One should avoid the use of the alkylating agent Melphalan in the induction phase of therapy where the plan is to proceed toward high-dose therapy with the same agent. The main reason for avoidance of the drug before mobilization lies in a decreased ability to achieve adequate numbers of CD34+ stem cells during apheresis. There appears to be a similar effect with prolonged use of lenalidomide before stem cell collection as well. As such, current International Myeloma Working Group consensus recommendations suggest no more than 4 cycles of lenalidomide-based therapy before stem cell mobilization.[171]

Although the diagnosis of myeloma can be made without a bone marrow evaluation, the procedure offers the only way to obtain a significant aliquot of plasma cells for full cytogenetic analysis. As mentioned previously, patients with multiple myeloma can be divided into risk categories based on routine cytogenetic and FISH analysis. Patients with high-risk cytogenetic lesions should be treated with a bortezomib-based chemotherapy regimen.

Options for bortezomib-based regimens in both the transplant- and nontransplant-eligible patients include bortezomib/lenalidomide/dexamethasone[172] and bortezomib/cyclophosphamide/dexamethasone (CyBorD).[173] These combinations are well tolerated and are associated with overall response rates of 80% to100%. The combination of bortezomib and dexamethasone alone, although very well tolerated, is associated with a lower overall response rate of 66%.[174]

Elderly patients with decreased performance status and a desire for a purely oral therapy have the option of lenalidomide and low-dose dexamethasone, which affords about a 70% overall response rate.[175] The use of thalidomide and dexamethasone is somewhat less attractive as an induction therapy not only because of the slightly lower response rates (overall response rate, 63%)[176] but also because of the side-effect profile, which includes peripheral neuropathy, gastrointestinal disturbance, somnolence, and thrombosis risk. The advantage of a thalidomide-based approach, however, lies in patients with diminished bone marrow reserve/function, as the drug is not associated with myelosuppression.

Any regimen that can be used in transplant-eligible patients can also be used in non–transplant-eligible patients as well. On the whole, the treatment paradigm has become a 2- or 3-drug regimen with a novel therapy and corticosteroid with and without a cytotoxic agent or 2 novel agents and corticosteroids. Although commonly used in Europe for nontransplant candidates, melphalan-based induction regimens are not used as frequently in the United States because of the availability of and activity/tolerability of novel therapies. The combination of melphalan and prednisone (MP) has been used for more than 50 years in clinical practice. before the advent of novel therapies, it was the cornerstone of management of non–transplant-eligible patients. It has been compared with the combination of melphalan, prednisone, and thalidomide (MPT) in numerous clinical trials. A recent meta-analysis concluded that although MPT versus MP results in a higher response rate (pooled odds ratio of 3.39 [$P<.001$]) and PFS (hazard ratio of 0.68 [$P<.001$]) there was only a nonstatistically significant trend toward improved OS (hazard ratio, 0.80 [$P=.07$]). These improvements came at the cost of significantly higher rates of thromboembolic events and higher degree of peripheral neuropathy.[177]

The presence of comorbid conditions and polypharmacy in elderly patients should help to guide therapy in scenarios in which multiple (otherwise equivalent) options exist. In addition, toxicity profile is key in selecting therapies. Drugs such as thalidomide and bortezomib may be difficult to administer in patients with baseline neuropathies from other conditions, such as diabetes. Agents such as lenalidomide and cyclophosphamide may be equally difficult in elderly patients with poor marrow reserve.

Renal dysfunction, although often associated with myeloma, is frequently seen in elderly patients for a variety of comorbid conditions, such as hypertension and diabetes. Agents such as bortezomib and cyclophosphamide can be administered at full doses, regardless of creatinine clearance; however, lenalidomide should be dose attenuated base on the degree of renal compromise.

Therapy in the Relapsed/Refractory Setting

Systemic therapy for elderly myeloma patients in the relapsed and refractory setting provides a variety of unique challenges. Considerations regarding optimal therapy in this setting include: (1) degree and duration of response to prior therapies, (2) toxicity profile, (3) tempo and type of relapse.

As many of the therapies utilized in the management of myeloma have synergy with one another, they can often be "re-used" in the relapsed setting in new combinations. A phase II trial evaluating the combination of lenalidomide, bortezomib, and dexamethasone in the relapsed/refractory setting, yielded a median OS of 26 months with 86% of patients alive at 1 year.[178]

Long-term follow-up data from the APEX trial (comparing bortezomib alone with high-dose dexamethasone) found a 43% response rate (CR+PR), a median OS of 29.8 months with 80% of patients alive at 1 year on the bortezomib arm.[179]

The combination of lenalidomide and dexamethasone is FDA approved for patients who have received at least 1 prior therapy. The approval stems from an article in the *New England Journal of Medicine* citing a 61% response rate (≥PR) with a median OS of 29.6 months.[180]

As in the upfront setting, the presence of comorbid conditions and toxicity profile plays an important role in the selection of appropriate therapy choices. Heavily pretreated patients may have significant therapy-induced peripheral neuropathy or bone marrow dysfunction. Therapies with nonoverlapping toxicities should be selected to maximize quality of life in the elderly population. Numerous regimens have been studied combining the agents listed above. Although some clinical trials do have age limitations, elderly patients with good performance status should be considered for experimental therapies.

Type and tempo of relapse should also factor into the decision for salvage therapies. Patients with long durations of remission after high-dose melphalan may be candidates for second transplants. Extensive visceral relapse of disease may warrant more aggressive approaches such as CyBorD. In very elderly and frail patients with serologic relapse only (no end-organ sequelae) risks and benefits of systemic therapy versus observation should be weighed carefully.

Supportive Care and Special Considerations

Thromboprophylaxis is germane to the treatment of elderly patients with myeloma. Compared with their aged-matched cohorts, patients with MGUS and MM, respectively, have a 3.3% and 9.2% relative risk of deep venous thrombosis.[181] Therapeutic use of immunomodulatory drug(s) (IMIds) are also associated with an increase in thromboembolic events, especially when used in conjunction with corticosteroids. These factors combined with a relative decline in mobility with age warrant diligent prophylaxis and treatment of blood clots. In addition, careful history and physical examinations are required during active therapy with a focused evaluation for signs and symptoms of deep venous thromboses and pulmonary emboli. The recommendation for patients receiving IMIds is prophylaxis with aspirin therapy with a consideration for low-molecular-weight heparin in patients with prior thromboembolic event or high risk for clot in the setting of multiple risk factors (ie, history of thromboembolic event, indwelling central venous catheter, inherited thrombophilia).[182] Posttransplant patients, as well as those receiving bortezomib-containing regimens are at a higher risk for varicella zoster virus reactivation and should undergo prophylaxis with antiviral therapy. In one study by Chanan-Khan and colleagues[183] the incidence of herpes zoster was 13%.

Continued efforts to balance efficacy in toxicity should be considered in the treatment of elderly patients with myeloma. Bortezomib-induced peripheral neuropathy can be quite debilitating in some patients, requiring cessation of the drug. New strategies have emerged in recent years in hopes of reducing the incidence of neuropathy without compromising efficacy. Two maneuvers that can be utilized are the subcutaneous administration of the drug as well as weekly dosing. In a randomized, phase

3 study, the subcutaneous administration of bortezomib was found to be noninferior to intravenous administration compounded by an improved safety profile.[184] Standard dosing of bortezomib on a 1, 4, 8, 11 schedule (every 21 days) has been compared with a weekly approach, and the latter is associated with a better safety profile with similar efficacy.[185]

Routine use of bisphosphonates, such as zoledronic acid and pamidronate, should be for patients with hypercalcemia or evidence of lytic bone disease. Skeletal events, such as compressions fractures, are a major source of morbidity and mortality in elderly patients with myeloma. Regular use of bisphosphonates have been found to reduce skeletal complications; however, the optimal dosing schedule for long-term bisphosphonate therapy is not entirely clear.[186] Given concern for osteonecrosis of the jaw, patients initiating therapy with bisphosphonates should have a complete dental evaluation. Ongoing clinical trials are evaluating the role of denosumab (a RANK ligand inhibitor recently FDA approved for management of bony disease in solid tumors) in patients with MM.

Symptomatic anemia stemming from disease progression or therapy-induced toxicity can plague patients with myeloma. Furthermore, elderly patients with long-standing cardiac disease may not be able to tolerate lower hemoglobin levels without a significant impact on quality of life. The use of erythropoietin-stimulating agents should be considered in elderly patients with myeloma. Consensus statements recommend starting at the lowest dose with plans to increase after 4 weeks if no response is seen. Erythropoietin-stimulating agents should be stopped after 6 to 8 weeks if there is no significant improvement in hemoglobin. Functional or true iron deficiency should be treated with supplemental intravenous iron.[187]

Future directions include new proteasome inhibitors, such as carfilzomib, and new IMIds, such as pomalidomide. Both of these agents have shown promising efficacy in the relapsed and refractory settings with tolerable side-effect profiles. Other avenues of research have focused on different exploitable pathways, such as mammalian target of rapamycin and histone deacytlase inhibition.

Conclusion

Multiple myeloma represents an incurable hematologic malignancy that primarily affects people of advanced age. Elderly people with signs of unexplained anemia, hypercalcemia, lytic bone disease, or renal dysfunction should be evaluated for this plasma cell dyscrasia. Full workup should include bone marrow evaluation (for cytogenetic profiling) and appropriate skeletal imaging. Eligibility for high-dose therapy and autologous stem cell transplantation should not be based solely on age and should incorporate performance status, disease status, and organ function. Choice of therapeutic combination should be sensitive to comorbid conditions and toxicity profile. Careful attention should be paid to the management of disease-related and treatment-related toxicities.

REFERENCES

1. Estey EH, Keating MJ, McCredie KB, et al. Causes of initial remission induction failure in acute myelogenous leukemia. Blood 1982;60(2):309–15.
2. Faderl S, Verstovsek S, Cortes J, et al. Clofarabine and cytarabine combination as induction therapy for acute myeloid leukemia (AML) in patients 50 years of age or older. Blood 2006;108(1):45–51.
3. Pollyea DA, Kohrt HE, Medeiros BC. Acute myeloid leukaemia in the elderly: a review. Br J Haematol 2011;152(5):524–42.

4. Juliusson G, Antunovic P, Derolf A, et al. Age and acute myeloid leukemia: real world data on decision to treat and outcomes from the Swedish Acute Leukemia Registry. Blood 2009;113(18):4179–87.
5. Byrd JC, Mrózek K, Dodge RK, et al. Pretreatment cytogenetic abnormalities are predictive of induction success, cumulative incidence of relapse, and overall survival in adult patients with de novo acute myeloid leukemia: results from Cancer and Leukemia Group B (CALGB 8461). Blood 2002;100(13):4325–36.
6. Slovak ML, Kopecky KJ, Cassileth PA, et al. Karyotypic analysis predicts outcome of preremission and postremission therapy in adult acute myeloid leukemia: a Southwest Oncology Group/Eastern Cooperative Oncology Group Study. Blood 2000; 96(13):4075–83.
7. Grimwade D, Hills RK, Moorman AV, et al. Refinement of cytogenetic classification in acute myeloid leukemia: determination of prognostic significance of rare recurring chromosomal abnormalities among 5876 younger adult patients treated in the United Kingdom Medical Research Council trials. Blood 2010;116(3):354–65.
8. Leith CP, Kopecky KJ, Godwin J, et al. Acute myeloid leukemia in the elderly: assessment of multidrug resistance (MDR1) and cytogenetics distinguishes biologic subgroups with remarkably distinct responses to standard chemotherapy. A Southwest Oncology Group study. Blood 1997;89(9):3323–9.
9. van der Holt B, Breems DA, Berna Beverloo H, et al. Various distinctive cytogenetic abnormalities in patients with acute myeloid leukaemia aged 60 years and older express adverse prognostic value: results from a prospective clinical trial. Br J Haematol 2007;136(1):96–105.
10. Bullinger L, Döhner K, Bair E, et al. Use of gene-expression profiling to identify prognostic subclasses in adult acute myeloid leukemia. N Engl J Med 2004;350(16): 1605–16.
11. Valk PJM, Verhaak RG, Beijen MA, et al. Prognostically useful gene-expression profiles in acute myeloid leukemia. N Engl J Med 2004;350(16):1617–28.
12. Rucker FG, Bullinger L, Schwaenen C, et al. Disclosure of candidate genes in acute myeloid leukemia with complex karyotypes using microarray-based molecular characterization. J Clin Oncol 2006;24(24):3887–94.
13. Haferlach T, Kohlmann A, Wieczorek L, et al. Clinical utility of microarray-based gene expression profiling in the diagnosis and subclassification of leukemia: report from the International Microarray Innovations in Leukemia Study Group. J Clin Oncol 2010;28(15):2529–37.
14. Marcucci G, Mrózek K, Radmacher MD, et al. The prognostic and functional role of microRNAs in acute myeloid leukemia. Blood 2011;117(4):1121–9.
15. Larson RA. Is modulation of multidrug resistance a viable strategy for acute myeloid leukemia? Leukemia 2003;17(3):488–91.
16. Baer MR, George SL, Dodge RK, et al. Phase 3 study of the multidrug resistance modulator PSC-833 in previously untreated patients 60 years of age and older with acute myeloid leukemia: Cancer and Leukemia Group B Study 9720. Blood 2002; 100(4):1224–32.
17. Cripe LD, Uno H, Paietta EM, et al. Zosuquidar, a novel modulator of P-glycoprotein, does not improve the outcome of older patients with newly diagnosed acute myeloid leukemia: a randomized, placebo-controlled trial of the Eastern Cooperative Oncology Group 3999. Blood 2010;116(20):4077–85.
18. Mayer RJ, Davis RB, Schiffer CA, et al. Intensive postremission chemotherapy in adults with acute myeloid leukemia. Cancer and Leukemia Group B. N Engl J Med 1994;331(14):896–903.

19. Lowenberg B, Suciu S, Archimbaud E, et al. Mitoxantrone versus daunorubicin in induction-consolidation chemotherapy—the value of low-dose cytarabine for maintenance of remission, and an assessment of prognostic factors in acute myeloid leukemia in the elderly: final report. European Organization for the Research and Treatment of Cancer and the Dutch-Belgian Hemato-Oncology Cooperative Hovon Group. J Clin Oncol 1998;16(3):872–81.

20. Wiernik PH, Banks PL, Case DC Jr, et al. Cytarabine plus idarubicin or daunorubicin as induction and consolidation therapy for previously untreated adult patients with acute myeloid leukemia. Blood 1992;79(2):313–9.

21. Ferrara F, Annunziata M, Copia C, et al. Therapeutic options and treatment results for patients over 75 years of age with acute myeloid leukemia. Haematologica 1998; 83(2):126–31.

22. Knipp S, Hildebrand B, Kündgen A, et al. Intensive chemotherapy is not recommended for patients aged >60 years who have myelodysplastic syndromes or acute myeloid leukemia with high-risk karyotypes. Cancer 2007;110(2):345–52.

23. Rowe JM, Neuberg D, Friedenberg W, et al. A phase 3 study of three induction regimens and of priming with GM-CSF in older adults with acute myeloid leukemia: a trial by the Eastern Cooperative Oncology Group. Blood 2004;103(2):479–85.

24. Lowenberg B, Ossenkoppele GJ, van Putten W, et al. High-dose daunorubicin in older patients with acute myeloid leukemia. [Erratum appears in N Engl J Med 2010;25;362(12):1155 Note: Dosage error in published abstract; MEDLINE/PubMed abstract corrected; Dosage error in article text]. N Engl J Med 2009; 361(13):1235–48.

25. Burnett AK, Milligan D, Goldstone A, et al. The impact of dose escalation and resistance modulation in older patients with acute myeloid leukaemia and high risk myelodysplastic syndrome: the results of the LRF AML14 trial. Br J Haematol 2009;145(3):318–32.

26. Schiller G, Lee M. Long-term outcome of high-dose cytarabine-based consolidation chemotherapy for older patients with acute myelogenous leukemia. Leukemia Lymphoma 1997;25(1–2):111–9.

27. Dombret H, Raffoux E, Gardin C. Acute myeloid leukemia in the elderly. Semin Oncol 2008;35(4):430–8.

28. Klepin HD, Balducci L. Acute myelogenous leukemia in older adults. Oncologist 2009;14(3):222–32.

29. Marks DI, Marks DI. Treating the "older" adult with acute lymphoblastic leukemia. Hematology 2010:1320.

30. Bertz H, Potthoff K, Finke J. Allogeneic stem-cell transplantation from related and unrelated donors in older patients with myeloid leukemia. J Clin Oncol 2003;21(8): 1480–4.

31. Valcarcel D, Martino R, Caballero D, et al. Sustained remissions of high-risk acute myeloid leukemia and myelodysplastic syndrome after reduced-intensity conditioning allogeneic hematopoietic transplantation: chronic graft-versus-host disease is the strongest factor improving survival. J Clin Oncol 2008;26(4):577–84.

32. Gyurkocza B, Storb R, Storer BE, et al. Nonmyeloablative allogeneic hematopoietic cell transplantation in patients with acute myeloid leukemia. J Clin Oncol 2010; 28(17):2859–67.

33. Farag SS, Archer KJ, Mrózek K, et al; Cancer and Leukemia Group B 8461. Pretreatment cytogenetics add to other prognostic factors predicting complete remission and long-term outcome in patients 60 years of age or older with acute myeloid leukemia: results from Cancer and Leukemia Group B 8461. Blood 2006; 108(1):63–73.

34. Rollig C, Thiede C, Gramatzki M, et al. A novel prognostic model in elderly patients with acute myeloid leukemia: results of 909 patients entered into the prospective AML96 trial. Blood 2010;116(6):971–8.

35. Wheatley K, Brookes CL, Howman AJ, et al. Prognostic factor analysis of the survival of elderly patients with AML in the MRC AML11 and LRF AML14 trials. Br J Haematol 2009;145(5):598–605.

36. Juliusson G, Swedish AMLG, Juliusson G. Most 70- to 79-year-old patients with acute myeloid leukemia do benefit from intensive treatment. Blood 2011;117(12):3473–4.

37. Burnett AK, Milligan D, Prentice AG, et al. A comparison of low-dose cytarabine and hydroxyurea with or without all-trans retinoic acid for acute myeloid leukemia and high-risk myelodysplastic syndrome in patients not considered fit for intensive treatment. Cancer 2007;109(6):1114–24.

38. Blum W, Garzon R, Klisovic RB, et al. Clinical response and miR-29b predictive significance in older AML patients treated with a 10-day schedule of decitabine. Proc Natl Acad Sci U S A 2010;107(16):7473–8.

39. Fenaux P, Mufti GJ, Hellstrom-Lindberg E, et al. Efficacy of azacitidine compared with that of conventional care regimens in the treatment of higher-risk myelodysplastic syndromes: a randomised, open-label, phase III study. Lancet Oncol 2009;10(3):223–32.

40. Green SR, Choudhary AK, Fleming IN. Combination of sapacitabine and HDAC inhibitors stimulates cell death in AML and other tumour types. Br J Cancer 2010;103(9):1391–9.

41. Prebet T, Vey N. Vorinostat in acute myeloid leukemia and myelodysplastic syndromes. Expert Opin Invest Drugs 2011;20(2):287–95.

42. Tickenbrock L, Klein HU, Trento C, et al. Increased HDAC1 deposition at hematopoietic promoters in AML and its association with patient survival. Leuk Res 2011;35(5):620–5.

43. Kantarjian H, Garcia-Manero G, O'Brien S, et al. Phase I clinical and pharmacokinetic study of oral sapacitabine in patients with acute leukemia and myelodysplastic syndrome. J Clin Oncol 2010;28(2):285–91.

44. Altman JK, Sassano A, Platanias LC. Targeting mTOR for the treatment of AML. New agents and new directions. Oncotarget 2011;2(6):510–7.

45. Tamburini J, Green AS, Chapuis N, et al. Targeting translation in acute myeloid leukemia: a new paradigm for therapy? Cell Cycle 2009;8(23):3893–9.

46. Fathi AT, Karp JE. New agents in acute myeloid leukemia: beyond cytarabine and anthracyclines. Curr Oncol Reports 2009;11(5):346–52.

47. Walsby EJ, Coles SJ, Knapper S, et al. The topoisomerase II inhibitor voreloxin causes cell cycle arrest and apoptosis in myeloid leukemia cells and acts in synergy with cytarabine. Haematologica 2011;96(3):393–9.

48. Zhu X, Ma Y. Liu D. Novel agents and regimens for acute myeloid leukemia: 2009 ASH annual meeting highlights. J Hematol Oncol 2010;3:17.

49. Knapper S, Burnett AK, Littlewood T, et al. A phase 2 trial of the FLT3 inhibitor lestaurtinib (CEP701) as first-line treatment for older patients with acute myeloid leukemia not considered fit for intensive chemotherapy. Blood 2006;108(10):3262–70.

50. Fehniger TA, Uy GL, Trinkaus K, et al. A phase 2 study of high-dose lenalidomide as initial therapy for older patients with acute myeloid leukemia. Blood 2011;117(6):182833.

51. Mato AR, Morgans AK, Luger SM. The generalized care of the patient with acute lymphoblastic leukemia. In: Advani AS, Lazarus HM, editors. Adult acute lymphocytic leukemia. Humana Press; 2011. p. 97–114.

52. Goldstone AH, Richards SM, Lazarus HM, et al. In adults with standard-risk acute lymphoblastic leukemia, the greatest benefit is achieved from a matched sibling allogeneic transplantation in first complete remission, and an autologous transplantation is less effective than conventional consolidation/maintenance chemotherapy in all patients: final results of the International ALL Trial (MRC UKALL XII/ECOG E2993). Blood 2008;111(4):1827–33.

53. Wetzler M, Sanford BL, Kurtzberg J, et al. Effective asparagine depletion with pegylated asparaginase results in improved outcomes in adult acute lymphoblastic leukemia: Cancer and Leukemia Group B Study 9511. Blood 2007;109(10):4164–7.

54. Larson RA, Dodge RK, Burns CP, et al. A five-drug remission induction regimen with intensive consolidation for adults with acute lymphoblastic leukemia: cancer and leukemia group B study 8811. Blood 1995;85(8):2025–37.

55. Chang JE, Medlin SC, Kahl BS, et al. Augmented and standard Berlin-Frankfurt-Munster chemotherapy for treatment of adult acute lymphoblastic leukemia. Leukemia Lymphoma 2008;49(12):2298–307.

56. Kantarjian H, Thomas D, O'Brien S, et al. Long-term follow-up results of hyperfractionated cyclophosphamide, vincristine, doxorubicin, and dexamethasone (Hyper-CVAD), a dose-intensive regimen, in adult acute lymphocytic leukemia. Cancer 2004;101(12):2788–801.

57. Earl M. Incidence and management of asparaginase-associated adverse events in patients with acute lymphoblastic leukemia. Clin Advance Hematol Oncol 2009;7(9):600–6.

58. Patel B, Richards SM, Rowe JM, et al. High incidence of avascular necrosis in adolescents with acute lymphoblastic leukaemia: a UKALL XII analysis. Leukemia 2008;22(2):308–12.

59. Fielding AK. Current treatment of Philadelphia chromosome-positive acute lymphoblastic leukemia. Haematologica 2010;95(1):8–12.

60. Ohno R. Changing paradigm of the treatment of Philadelphia chromosome-positive acute lymphoblastic leukemia. Curr Hematol Malignancy Rep 2010;5(4):213–21.

61. Ohno R, Japan Adult Leukemia Study, Treatment of Philadelphia-chromosome-positive acute lymphoblastic leukemia with imatinib in combination with chemotherapy. Curr Hematol Malignancy Reports 2006;1(3):180–7.

62. Ottmann OG, Wassmann B. Treatment of Philadelphia chromosome-positive acute lymphoblastic leukemia. Hematology:118–22.

63. Ravandi F, O'Brien S, Thomas D, et al. First report of phase 2 study of dasatinib with hyper-CVAD for the frontline treatment of patients with Philadelphia chromosome-positive (Ph+) acute lymphoblastic leukemia. Blood 2010;116(12):2070–7.

64. Vignetti M, Fazi P, Cimino G, et al. Imatinib plus steroids induces complete remissions and prolonged survival in elderly Philadelphia chromosome-positive patients with acute lymphoblastic leukemia without additional chemotherapy: results of the Gruppo Italiano Malattie Ematologiche dell'Adulto (GIMEMA) LAL0201-B protocol. Blood 2007;109(9):3676–8.

65. Ottmann O, Dombret H, Martinelli G, et al. Dasatinib induces rapid hematologic and cytogenetic responses in adult patients with Philadelphia chromosome positive acute lymphoblastic leukemia with resistance or intolerance to imatinib: interim results of a phase 2 study. Blood 2007;110(7):2309–15.

66. Marks DI, Pérez WS, He W, et al. Unrelated donor transplants in adults with Philadelphia-negative acute lymphoblastic leukemia in first complete remission. Blood 2008;112(2):426–34.

67. Bartolozzi B, Bosi A, Orsi C. Allogeneic hematopoietic stem cell transplantation as part of postremission therapy improves survival for adult patients with high-risk acute lymphoblastic leukemia: a meta-analysis. Cancer 2007;109(2):343 [author reply: 344].

68. Bachanova V, Verneris MR, DeFor T, et al. Prolonged survival in adults with acute lymphoblastic leukemia after reduced-intensity conditioning with cord blood or sibling donor transplantation. Blood 2009;113(13):2902–5.

69. Marks DI, Wang T, Pérez WS, et al. The outcome of full-intensity and reduced-intensity conditioning matched sibling or unrelated donor transplantation in adults with Philadelphia chromosome-negative acute lymphoblastic leukemia in first and second complete remission. Blood 2010;116(3):366–74.

70. Mohty M, Labopin M, Volin L, et al. Reduced-intensity versus conventional myeloablative conditioning allogeneic stem cell transplantation for patients with acute lymphoblastic leukemia: a retrospective study from the European Group for Blood and Marrow Transplantation. Blood 2010;116(22):4439–43.

71. Fielding AK, Richards SM, Chopra R, et al. Outcome of 609 adults after relapse of acute lymphoblastic leukemia (ALL); an MRC UKALL12/ECOG 2993 study. Blood 2007;109(3):944–50.

72. Tavernier E, Boiron JM, Huguet F, et al. Outcome of treatment after first relapse in adults with acute lymphoblastic leukemia initially treated by the LALA-94 trial. Leukemia 21(9):190714.

73. DeAngelo DJ. Nelarabine for the treatment of patients with relapsed or refractory T-cell acute lymphoblastic leukemia or lymphoblastic lymphoma. Hematolo Oncol Clin North Am 2009;23(5):1121–35, vii–viii.

74. DeAngelo DJ, Yu D, Johnson JL, et al. Nelarabine induces complete remissions in adults with relapsed or refractory T-lineage acute lymphoblastic leukemia or lymphoblastic lymphoma: Cancer and Leukemia Group B study 19801. Blood 2007; 109(12):5136–42.

75. Larson RA. Three new drugs for acute lymphoblastic leukemia: nelarabine, clofarabine, and forodesine. Semin Oncol 2007;34(6 Suppl 5):S13–20.

76. Nijmeijer BA, van Schie ML, Halkes CJ, et al. A mechanistic rationale for combining alemtuzumab and rituximab in the treatment of ALL. Blood 2010;116(26):5930–40.

77. Thomas DA. Rituximab as therapy for acute lymphoblastic leukemia. Clin Advance Hematol Oncol 2010;8(3):168–71.

78. Thomas DA, O'Brien S, Faderl S, et al. Chemoimmunotherapy with a modified hyper-CVAD and rituximab regimen improves outcome in de novo Philadelphia chromosome-negative precursor B-lineage acute lymphoblastic leukemia. J Clin Oncol 2010;28(24):3880–9.

79. Angiolillo AL, Yu AL, Reaman G, et al. A phase II study of Campath-1H in children with relapsed or refractory acute lymphoblastic leukemia: a Children's Oncology Group report. Pediatr Blood Cancer 2009;53(6):978–83.

80. Parnes A, Bifulco C, Vanasse GJ. A novel regimen incorporating the concomitant administration of fludarabine and alemtuzumab for the treatment of refractory adult acute lymphoblastic leukaemia: a report of three cases. Br J Haematol 2007;139(1): 164–5.

81. Tibes R, Keating MJ, Ferrajoli A, et al. Activity of alemtuzumab in patients with CD52-positive acute leukemia. Cancer 2006;106(12):2645–51.

82. Dijoseph JF, Dougher MM, Armellino DC, et al. Therapeutic potential of CD22-specific antibody-targeted chemotherapy using inotuzumab ozogamicin (CMC-544) for the treatment of acute lymphoblastic leukemia. Leukemia 2007;21(11):2240–5.

83. Avellino R, Romano S, Parasole R, et al. Rapamycin stimulates apoptosis of childhood acute lymphoblastic leukemia cells. Blood 2005;106(4):1400–6.

84. Chiarini F, Falà F, Tazzari PL, et al. Dual inhibition of class IA phosphatidylinositol 3-kinase and mammalian target of rapamycin as a new therapeutic option for T-cell acute lymphoblastic leukemia. Cancer Res 2009;69(8):3520–8.

85. Chiarini F, Grimaldi C, Ricci F, et al. Activity of the novel dual phosphatidylinositol 3-kinase/mammalian target of rapamycin inhibitor NVP-BEZ235 against T-cell acute lymphoblastic leukemia. Cancer Res 2010;70(20):8097–107.

86. Guo D, Teng Q, Ji C. NOTCH and phosphatidylinositide 3-kinase/phosphatase and tensin homolog deleted on chromosome ten/AKT/mammalian target of rapamycin (mTOR) signaling in T-cell development and T-cell acute lymphoblastic leukemia. Leukemia Lymphoma 2011;52(7):1200–10.

87. Hirase C, Maeda Y, Takai S, et al. Hypersensitivity of Ph-positive lymphoid cell lines to rapamycin: possible clinical application of mTOR inhibitor. Leukemia Res 2009; 33(3):450–9.

88. Saunders P, Cisterne A, Weiss J, et al. The mammalian target of rapamycin inhibitor RAD001 (everolimus) synergizes with chemotherapeutic agents, ionizing radiation and proteasome inhibitors in pre-B acute lymphocytic leukemia. Haematologica 2011;96(1):69–77.

89. Li X, Gounari F, Protopopov A, et al. Oncogenesis of T-ALL and nonmalignant consequences of overexpressing intracellular NOTCH1. J Exp Med 2008;205(12):2851–61.

90. Beesley AH, Palmer ML, Ford J, et al. In vitro cytotoxicity of nelarabine, clofarabine and flavopiridol in paediatric acute lymphoblastic leukaemia. Br J Haematol 2007; 137(2):109–16.

91. Jackman KM, Frye CB, Hunger SP. Flavopiridol displays preclinical activity in acute lymphoblastic leukemia. Pediatr Blood Cancer 2008;50(4):772–8.

92. Karp JE, Passaniti A, Gojo I, et al. Phase I and pharmacokinetic study of flavopiridol followed by 1-beta-D-arabinofuranosylcytosine and mitoxantrone in relapsed and refractory adult acute leukemias. Clin Cancer Res 2005;11(23):8403–12.

93. Karp JE, Ross DD, Yang W, et al. Timed sequential therapy of acute leukemia with flavopiridol: in vitro model for a phase I clinical trial. Clin Cancer Res 2003;9(1):307–15.

94. Talarico L, Chen G, Pazdur R. Enrollment of elderly patients in clinical trials for cancer drug registration: a 7-year experience by the US Food and Drug Administration. J Clin Oncol 2004;22(22):4626–31.

95. Repetto L, Fratino L, Audisio RA, et al. Comprehensive Geriatric Assessment Adds Information to Eastern Cooperative Oncology Group Performance Status in Elderly Cancer Patients: An Italian Group for Geriatric Oncology Study. J Clinl Oncol 2002;20(2):494–502.

96. Luciani A, Ascione G, Bertuzzi C, et al. Detecting disabilities in older patients with cancer: comparison between Comprehensive Geriatric Assessment and Vulnerable Elders Survey-13. J Clin Oncol 2010;28(12):2046–50.

97. Charlson ME, Pompei P, Ales KL, MacKenzie CR. A new method of classifying prognostic comorbidity in longitudinal studies: development and validation. J Chronic Dis 1987;40(5):373.

98. Wedding U, Roehrig B, Klippstein A, et al. Comorbidity in patients with cancer: prevalence and severity measured by cumulative illness rating scale. Crit Rev Oncol Hematol 2007;61(3):269–76.

99. Hurria A, Gupta S, Zauderer M, et al. Developing a cancer-specific geriatric assessment. Cancer, 2005;104(9):1998–2005.

100. Siegel A, Lachs M, Coleman M, et al. Lymphoma in elderly patients: novel functional assessment techniques provide better discrimination among patients than traditional performance status measures. Clin Lymphoma, Myeloma Leukemia 2006;7(1):65–9.

101. Evens AM, Nabhan C, Helenowski I, et al. Multicenter Analysis of 150 very elderly non-hodgkin's lymphoma (nhl) patients: impact of comorbidities and response to initial therapy on survival. Blood (ASH Annual Meeting Abstracts) 2010;116:Abstract 3124.

102. Alizadeh AA, Eisen MB, Davis RE. Distinct types of diffuse large B-cell lymphoma identified by gene expression. Nature 2000;403:503–11.

103. Compagno M, Grunn A, Nandula SV, et al. Mutations of multiple genes cause deregulation of NF-kappaB in diffuse large B-cell lymphoma. Nature 2009; 459(7247):717.

104. Davis RE, Ngo V, Lenz G, et al. Chronic active B-cell-receptor signalling in diffuse large B-cell lymphoma. Nature 2010;463(7277):88.

105. Monti S, Savage K, Kutok JL, et al. Molecular profiling of diffuse large B-cell lymphoma identifies robust subtypes including one characterized by host inflammatory response. Blood 2005;105(5):1851.

106. Hans CP, Weisenburger DD, Greiner TC, et al. Confirmation of the miolecular classification of diffuse large B-cell lymphoma by immunohistochemistry using a tissue microarray. Blood 2004;103(1):275.

107. Savage KJ, Johnson NA, Ben-Neriah S, et al. MYC gene rearrangement are associated with a poor porgosis in ndiffuse large B-cell lymphoma patients treated with R-CHOP chemotherapy. Blood 2009;114(17):3533.

108. Park S, Lee J, Ko YH, et al. The impact of Epstein-Barr virus status on clinical outcome in diffuse large B-cell lymphoma. Blood 2007;110(3):972.

109. Ziepert M, Hasenclever D, Kuhnt E, et al. Standard International Prognostic Index remains a valid predictor of outcome for patients with aggressive CD20+ B-cell lymphoma in the rituximab era. J Clin Oncol 2010;28(14):2373–80.

110. Pfreundschuh M. How I treat elderly patients with diffuse large B-cell lymphoma. Blood 2010;116(24):5103–10.

111. Tucci A, Bottelli C, Ferrari S, et al. A comprehensive geriatric assessment is more effective than clinical judgement to prospectively identify elderly patients with diffuse large cell lymphoma who can tolerate full-dose anthracyclin-based treatment and achieve the same outcome as young patients. Blood (ASH Annual Meeting Abstracts) 2007;110(11):Abstract 3441.

112. Tirelli U, Fratino L, Balzarotti M, et al. Comprehensive Geriatric assessment-adapted chemotherapy in elderly patients (>70 years) with diffuse large B-cell non-Hodgkin's lymphoma (DLBCL): final results and long term follow-up. Blood (ASH Annual Meeting Abstracts) 2009;114(22):Abstract 2684.

113. Coiffier B, Lepage E, Briere J, et al. CHOP Chemotherapy plus Rituximab compared with CHOP alone in Elderly patients with diffuse large-B-cell lymphoma. N Engl J Med 2002;346(4):235–42.

114. Feugier P, Van Hoof A, Sebban C, et al. Long-term results of the R-CHOP Study in the treatment of elderly patients with diffuse large B-cell lymphoma: a study by the Groupe d'Etude des Lymphomes de l'Adulte. J Clin Oncol 2005;23(18):4117–26.

115. Pfreundschuh M, Schubert J, Ziepert M, et al. Six vs. eight cycles of bi-weekly CHOP-14 with or without Rituximab for elderly patients with diffuse large b-cell lymphoma (dlbcl): results of the completed RICOVER-60 Trial of the German High-Grade Non-Hodgkin Lymphoma Study Group (DSHNHL). Blood (ASH Annual Meeting Abstracts) 2006;108(11):Abstract 205.

116. Pfreundschuh M, Ziepert M, Reiser M, et al. The role of radiotherapy to bulky disease in the rituximab era: results from two prospective trials of the German High-Grade Non-Hodgkin- Lymphoma Study Group (DSHNHL) for elderly patients with DLBCL. Blood (ASH Annual Meeting Abstracts) 2008;112(11):Abstract 584.

117. Habermann TM, Weller EA, Morrison VA, et al. Rituximab-CHOP versus CHOP alone or with maintenance rituximab in older patients with diffuse large B-cell lymphoma. J Clin Oncol 2006; 24(19):3121–7.

118. Philip T, Guglielmi C, Hagenbeek A, et al. Autologous bone marrow transplantation as compared with salvage chemotherapy in relapses of chemotherapy-sensitive non-Hodgkin's lymphoma. N Engl J Med 1995;333(23):1540–5.

119. Gisselbrecht C, Glass B, Mounier N, et al. Salvage regimens with autologous transplantation for relapsed large B-cell lymphoma in the rituximab era. J Clin Oncol 2010;28(27):4184–90.

120. Elstrom R, Martin P, Rua SH, et al. Autologous stem cell transplantation is feasible and of potential benefit in very elderly patients with lymphoma and limited comorbidities. Blood (ASH Annual Meeting Abstracts) 2010;116(21):Abstract 3561.

121. Koreth J, Aldridge J, Kim HT, et al. Reduced-intensity conditioning hematopoietic stem cell transplantation in patients over 60 years: hematologic malignancy outcomes are not impaired in advanced age. Biology of Blood and Marrow Transplantation: Journal of the American Society for Blood and Marrow Transplantation 2010;16(6):792–800.

122. Rupolo M, Michieli M, Spina M, et al. High dose therapy (HDCT) with autologous stem cell transplantation (ASCT) for non-Hodgkin lymphoma in the elderly: feasibility of a patient-tailored treatment plan. Blood (ASH Annual Meeting Abstracts) 2004; 104(11):Abstract 5216.

123. Wildes TM, Augustin KM, Sempek D, et al. Comorbidities, not age, impact outcomes in autologous stem cell transplant for relapsed non-hodgkin lymphoma. Biology of Blood and Marrow Transplantation: Journal of the American Society for Blood and Marrow Transplantation 2008;14(7):840–6.

124. Wildes TM, Augustin KM, Vij R, et al. Comparison of outcomes in elderly patients with non-Hodgkins lymphoma undergoing high-dose chemotherapy to their younger counterparts: greater morbidity but no significant impact on overall survival. Blood (ASH Annual Meeting Abstracts) 2005;106(11):Abstract 2086.

125. Hamlin PA, Alma RM, Portlock NA, et al. Final results of a phase II study of sequential R-CHOP and yttrium-90 ibritumomab tiuxetan (RIT) for elderly high risk patients with untreated diffuse large B-cell lymphoma (DLBCL). Blood (ASH Annual Meeting Abstracts) 2010;116(21):Abstract 1793.

126. Zinzani PL, Tani M, Fanti S, et al. A phase II trial of CHOP chemotherapy followed by yttrium 90 (90Y) ibritumomab tiuxetan (Zevalin) for Previously untreated elderly diffuse large B-cell lymphoma (DLBCL) patients. Blood (ASH Annual Meeting Abstracts) 2005;106(11):Abstract 4765.

127. Boehme V, Schmitz N, Zeynalova S, et al. CNS events in elderly patients with aggressive lymphoma treated with modern chemotherapy (CHOP-14) with or without rituximab: an analysis of patients treated in the RICOVER-60 trial of the German High-Grade Non-Hodgkin Lymphoma Study Group (DSHNHL). Blood 2009; 113(17):3896–902.

128. Oyama T, Ichimura K, Suzuki R, et al. Senile EBV+ B-cell lymphoproliferative disorders: a clinicopathologic study of 22 patients. Am J Surg Pathol 2003;27(1): 16–26.

129. Gibson SE, Hsi ED. Epstein-Barr virus–positive B-cell lymphoma of the elderly at a United States tertiary medical center: an uncommon aggressive lymphoma with a nongerminal center B-cell phenotype. Hum Pathol 2009;40(5):653–61.

130. Hoeller S, Tzankov A, Pileri SA, et al. Epstein-Barr virus-positive diffuse large B-cell lymphoma in elderly patients is rare in Western populations. Hum Pathol 2010;41(3): 352–7.

131. Abrey LE, Batchelor TT, Ferreri AJ, et al. Report of an international workshop to standardize baseline evaluation and response criteria for primary CNS lymphoma. J Clin Oncol 2005;23(22):5034.

132. Ney DE, Reiner AS, Panageas KS, et al. Characteristics and outcomes of elderly patients with primary central nervous system lymphoma. Cancer 2010;116(19): 4605–12.

133. Gerstner ER, Carson KA, Grossman SA, et al. Long-term outcome in PCNSL patients treated with high-dose methotrexate and deferred radiation. Neurology 2008;70(5):401.

134. Zhu JJ, Gerstner ER, Engler DA, et al. High-dose methotrexate for elderly patients with primary CNS lymphoma. Neuro Oncol 2008;11(2):211–5.

135. Ferreri AJ, Reni M, Foppoli M, et al. High-dose cytarabine plus high-dose methotrexate versus high-dose methotrexate alone in patients with primary CNS lymphoma: a randomised phase 2 trial. Lancet 2009;374(9700):1512–20.

136. Rubenstein JL, Johnson JL, Jung SH, et al. Intensive chemotherapy and immunotherapy, without brain irradiation, in newly diagnosed patients with primary CNS lymphoma: Results of CALGB 50202. Blood (ASH Annual Meeting Abstracts) 2010;116(21):Abstract 763.

137. Enting RH, Demopoulos A, DeAngelis LM, et al. Salvage therapy for primary CNS lymphoma with a combination of rituximab and temozolomide. Neurology 2004; 64(5):934.

138. Voloschin A, Betensky R, Wen PY, et al. Topotecan as salvage therapy for relapsed or refractory primary central nervous system lymphoma. J Neuro-Oncol 2008;86(2): 211–5.

139. Engert A, Ballova V, Haverkamp H, et al. Hodgkin's lymphoma in elderly patients: a comprehensive retrospective analysis from the German Hodgkin's Study Group. J Clin Oncol 2005;23(22):5052–60.

140. Klimm B, Eich HT, Haverkamp H, et al. Poorer outcome of elderly patients treated with extended-field radiotherapy compared with involved-field radiotherapy after chemotherapy for Hodgkin's lymphoma: an analysis from the German Hodgkin Study Group. Ann Oncol 2007;18(2):357–63.

141. Chen R, Smith SE, Ansell SM, et al. Results of a pivotal phase 2 study of brentuximab vedotin (sgn-35) in patients with relapsed or refractory Hodgkin lymphoma. Blood 2010;116: Abstract 283.

142. Solal-Céligny P, Roy P, Colombat P, et al. Follicular Lymphoma International Prognostic Index. Blood 2004;104(5):1258–65.

143. Federico M, Bellei M, Marcheselli L, et al. Follicular Lymphoma International Prognostic Index 2: a new prognostic index for follicular lymphoma developed by the International Follicular Lymphoma Prognostic Factor Project. J Clin Oncol 2009; 27(27):4555–62.

144. Advani R, Rosenberg SA, Horning SJ. Stage I and II follicular non-Hodgkin's lymphoma: long-term follow-up of no initial therapy. J Clin Oncol 2004;22(8): 1454–9.

145. Hainsworth JD, Litchy M, Burris HA 3rd, et al. Rituximab as First-line and maintenance therapy for patients with indolent non-Hodgkin's lymphoma. J Clin Oncol 2002;20(20):4261–7.

146. Colombat P, Salles G, Brousse N, et al. Rituximab (anti-CD20 monoclonal antibody) as single first-line therapy for patients with follicular lymphoma with a low tumor burden: clinical and molecular evaluation. Blood 2001;97(1):101–6.

147. Buske C, Kneba M, Lengfelder E, et al. Front-line combined immuno-chemotherapy (R-CHOP) significantly improves the time to treatment failure and overall survival in elderly patients with advanced stage follicular lymphoma—results of a prospective randomized trial of the German Low Grade Lymphoma Study Group (GLSG). Blood (ASH Annual Meeting Abstracts) 2006;108(11):Abstract 482.

148. Rummel MJ, Niederle N, Maschmeyer G, et al. Bendamustine Plus rituximab is superior in respect of progression free survival and cr rate when compared to CHOP plus rituximab as first-line treatment of patients with advanced follicular, indolent, and mantle cell lymphomas: final results of a randomized phase III study of the StiL (Study Group Indolent Lymphomas, Germany). Blood (Annual Meeting abstracts) 2009;114:Abstract 405.

149. Salles GA, Seymour JF, Feugier P, et al. Rituximab maintenance for 2 years in patients with untreated high tumor burden follicular lymphoma after response to immunochemotherapy. Asco Annual meeting, 2010: Abstract 8004.

150. Morschhauser F, Bischof-Delaloye A, Rohatiner AZS, et al. Extended follow-up of the International Randomized Phase 3 First-Line Indolent Trial (FIT) shows durable benefit of 90 y-ibritumomab tiuxetan (zevalin(r)) consolidation of first remission in advanced stage follicular non-Hodgkin's lymphoma. Blood (Annual Meeting Abstracts) 2008;112:Abstract 2002.

151. Jemal A, Siegel R, Xu J, et al. Cancer statistics, 2010. CA Cancer J Clin 2010;60(5): 277–300.

152. Rajkumar SV, Kyle RA. Multiple myeloma: diagnosis and treatment. Mayo Clin Proc 2005;80(10):1371–82.

153. Kyle RA, Therneau TM, Rajkumar SV, et al. Prevalence of monoclonal gammopathy of undetermined significance. N Engl J Med 2006;354(13):1362–9.

154. Rajkumar SV, Kyle RA, Therneau TM, et al. Serum free light chain ratio is an independent risk factor for progression in monoclonal gammopathy of undetermined significance. Blood 2005;106(3):812–7.

155. Blade J, Dimopoulos M, Rosiñol L, et al. Smoldering (asymptomatic) multiple myeloma: current diagnostic criteria, new predictors of outcome, and follow-up recommendations. J Clin Oncol 2010;28(4):690–7.

156. Durie BG, Salmon SE. A clinical staging system for multiple myeloma. Correlation of measured myeloma cell mass with presenting clinical features, response to treatment, and survival. Cancer 1975;36(3):842–54.

157. Greipp PR, San Miguel J, Durie BG, et al. International staging system for multiple myeloma. J Clin Oncol, 2005. 23(15): p. 3412–20.

158. Kumar SK, Mikhael JR, Buadi FK, et al. Management of newly diagnosed symptomatic multiple myeloma: updated Mayo Stratification of Myeloma and Risk-Adapted Therapy (mSMART) consensus guidelines. Mayo Clin Proc 2009;84(12):1095–110.

159. Howlader N, Noone AM, Krapcho M, et al, editors. SEER Cancer Statistics Review, 1975–2008, National Cancer Institute. Bethesda, MD. Available at: http://seer.cancer.gov/csr/1975_2008/.

160. Abdelkefi A, Ladeb S, Torjman L, et al. Single autologous stem-cell transplantation followed by maintenance therapy with thalidomide is superior to double autologous transplantation in multiple myeloma: results of a multicenter randomized clinical trial. Blood 2008;111(4):1805–10.

161. To LB, Shepperd KM, Haylock DN, et al. Single high doses of cyclophosphamide enable the collection of high numbers of hemopoietic stem cells from the peripheral blood. Exp Hematol 1990;18(5): 442–7.

162. Jantunen E, Putkonen M, Nousiainen T, et al. Low-dose or intermediate-dose cyclophosphamide plus granulocyte colony-stimulating factor for progenitor cell mobilisation in patients with multiple myeloma. Bone Marrow Transplant 2003;31(5): 347–51.

163. Lazzarino M, Corso A, Barbarano L, et al. DCEP (dexamethasone, cyclophosphamide, etoposide, and cisplatin) is an effective regimen for peripheral blood stem cell collection in multiple myeloma. Bone Marrow Transplant 2001;28(9):835–9.

164. Majolino I, Marcenò R, Buscemi F, et al. Mobilization of circulating progenitor cells in multiple myeloma during VCAD therapy with or without rhG-CSF. Haematologica 1995;80(2):108–14.

165. Lefrere F, Zohar S, Ghez D, et al. The VAD chemotherapy regimen plus a G-CSF dose of 10 microg/kg is as effective and less toxic than high-dose cyclophosphamide plus a G-CSF dose of 5 microg/kg for progenitor cell mobilization: results from a monocentric study of 82 patients. Bone Marrow Transplant 2006;37(8):725–9.

166. Barlogie B, Anaissie E, van Rhee F, et al. Incorporating bortezomib into upfront treatment for multiple myeloma: early results of total therapy 3. Br J Haematol 2007;138(2):176–85.

167. Morris CL, Siegel E, Barlogie B, et al. Mobilization of CD34+ cells in elderly patients (>/= 70 years) with multiple myeloma: influence of age, prior therapy, platelet count and mobilization regimen. Br J Haematol 2003;120(3):413–23.

168. DiPersio JF, Stadtmauer EA, Nademanee A, et al. Plerixafor and G-CSF versus placebo and G-CSF to mobilize hematopoietic stem cells for autologous stem cell transplantation in patients with multiple myeloma. Blood 2009;113(23):5720–6.

169. Palumbo A, Bringhen S, Bruno B, et al. Melphalan 200 mg/m(2) versus melphalan 100 mg/m(2) in newly diagnosed myeloma patients: a prospective, multicenter phase 3 study. Blood 2010; 115(10):1873–9.

170. Bashir Q, Shah N, Parmar S, et al. Feasibility of autologous hematopoietic stem cell transplant in patients aged >/=70 years with multiple myeloma. Leuk Lymphoma 2011.

171. Kumar S, Giralt S, Stadtmauer EA, et al. Mobilization in myeloma revisited: IMWG consensus perspectives on stem cell collection following initial therapy with thalidomide-, lenalidomide-, or bortezomib-containing regimens. Blood 2009;114(9):1729–35.

172. Richardson PG, Weller E, Lonial S, et al. Lenalidomide, bortezomib, and dexamethasone combination therapy in patients with newly diagnosed multiple myeloma. Blood 2010;116(5):679–86.

173. Reeder CB, Reece DE, Kukreti V, et al. Cyclophosphamide, bortezomib and dexamethasone induction for newly diagnosed multiple myeloma: high response rates in a phase II clinical trial. Leukemia 2009;23(7):1337–41.

174. Harousseau JL, Attal M, Leleu X, et al. Bortezomib plus dexamethasone as induction treatment prior to autologous stem cell transplantation in patients with newly diagnosed multiple myeloma: results of an IFM phase II study. Haematologica 2006;91(11):1498–505.

175. Rajkumar SV, Jacobus S, Callander NS, et al. Lenalidomide plus high-dose dexamethasone versus lenalidomide plus low-dose dexamethasone as initial therapy for newly diagnosed multiple myeloma: an open-label randomised controlled trial. Lancet Oncol 2010;11(1):29–37.

176. Rajkumar SV, Blood E, Vesole D, et al. Phase III clinical trial of thalidomide plus dexamethasone compared with dexamethasone alone in newly diagnosed multiple myeloma: a clinical trial coordinated by the Eastern Cooperative Oncology Group. J Clin Oncol 2006;24(3):431–6.

177. Kapoor P, Rajkumar SV, Dispenzieri A, et al. Melphalan and prednisone versus melphalan, prednisone and thalidomide for elderly and/or transplant ineligible patients with multiple myeloma: a meta-analysis. Leukemia 2011;25(4): 689–96.

178. Richardson PG, Jagannath S, Jakubowiak AJ, et al. Phase II trial of lenalidomide, bortezomib, and dexamethasone in patiens with relapsed and relapsed/refractory multiple myeloma: updated efficacy and safety data after > 2 years of follow-up. Blood (ASH Annual Meeting Abstracts);116:Abstract 3049.

179. Richardson PG, Sonneveld P, Schuster M, et al. Extended follow-up of a phase 3 trial in relapsed multiple myeloma: final time-to-event results of the APEX trial. Blood 2007;110(10):3557–60.

180. Weber DM, Chen C, Niesvizky R, et al. Lenalidomide plus dexamethasone for relapsed multiple myeloma in North America. N Engl J Med 2007; 357(21):2133–42.

181. Kristinsson SY, Fears TR, Gridley G, et al. Deep vein thrombosis after monoclonal gammopathy of undetermined significance and multiple myeloma. Blood 2008; 112(9):3582–6.

182. Palumbo A, Rajkumar SV, Dimopoulos MA, et al. Prevention of thalidomide- and lenalidomide-associated thrombosis in myeloma. Leukemia 2008;22(2):414–23.

183. Chanan-Khan A, Sonneveld P, Schuster MW, et al. Analysis of herpes zoster events among bortezomib-treated patients in the phase III APEX study. J Clin Oncol 2008;26(29):4784–90.

184. Moreau P, Pylypenko H, Grosicki S, et al. Subcutaneous versus intravenous administration of bortezomib in patients with relapsed multiple myeloma: a randomised, phase 3, non-inferiority study. Lancet Oncol 2011;12(5):431–40.

185. Bringhen S, Larocca A, Rossi D, et al. Efficacy and safety of once-weekly bortezomib in multiple myeloma patients. Blood 2010;116(23):4745–53.

186. Berenson JR, Hillner BE, Kyle RA, et al. American Society of Clinical Oncology clinical practice guidelines: the role of bisphosphonates in multiple myeloma. J Clin Oncol 2002;20(17):3719–36.

187. Snowden JA, Ahmedzai SH, Ashcroft J, et al. Guidelines for supportive care in multiple myeloma 2011. Br J Haematol 2011;154(1):76–103.

Index

Note: Page numbers of article titles are in **boldface** type.

A

Abiraterone, 10
Activities of daily living, dependence in, and cancer, 5
Age, and cancer, general considerations, **1–18**
  increasing incidence of cancer with, 2
Aging, and cancer, 94–95
  physiologic changes with, 35, 36
Androgen deprivation, in metastatic prostate cancer, 10
Aromatase inhibitors, in breast cancer, 78
Axillary lymph node dissection, 54–55

B

B-cell neoplasms, mature, WHO 2008, 122–123
Bevacizumab, 43
Biological therapy, 11
Bisphosphonates, 44
  in myeloma, 140
Bladder cancer, 41
  clinically localized muscle-invasive, 41
  metastatic, 41
Body composition changes, and cancer incidence, 3
Bortezomib, in myeloma, 139–140
Breast cancer, 53–55
  biology of, in older woman, 73–74
  early, in older woman, **73–91**
  endocrine therapy in, 78–79
  follow-up of older woman with, 81–83
  incidence and mortality of, by age, 73
  metastatic, age and, 4
  outcome studies of, 53, 54
  treatment of, cardiac side effects of, 82–83
    chemotherapy in, 79–81
    constitutional side effects of, 81–82
    patterns in, 74–75
    radiation therapy in, 76–77
    recommendations for, 55
    skeletal side effects of, 83
    surgical, 75–76
    systemic therapy in, 77–81
Burkitt's lymphoma, treatment of, 127–128

Clin Geriatr Med 28 (2012) 153–157
doi:10.1016/S0749-0690(12)00020-1
0749-0690/12/$ – see front matter © 2012 Elsevier Inc. All rights reserved.

geriatric.theclinics.com